THE
HYPERACTIVE CHILD
AND THE FAMILY

THE
HYPERACTIVE
CHILD
AND
THE FAMILY

THE COMPLETE WHAT-TO-DO HANDBOOK

John F. Taylor, Ph.D.

FOREWORD BY
Thomas N. Fairchild, Ph.D.

Publishers Everest House *New York*

FEB

1981

Library of Congress Cataloging in Publication Data:
Taylor, John F   1944-
  The hyperactive child and the family.
  Includes index.
    1. Hyperactive children.   I. Title.
  RJ 506.H9T38   1980   618.92'8589   79-56871
  ISBN: 0-89696-080-3

Published simultaneously in Canada by
Beaverbooks, Pickering, Ontario

Printed in the United States of America

Designed by Joyce Cameron Weston
2RRD980

*To all hyperactive children and adults
and their brothers, sisters,
and parents*

Contents

7

8   CONTENTS

Acknowledgments

The ultimate test of any guidebook is whether it works in the lives of those whom it is intended to help. Eleven parents of hyperactive children, each of whom has actively helped other such parents, reviewed portions of the manuscript and gave suggestions for increasing its effectiveness. These parents are Chris Chapin, Joy Guerber, Mary Jo Hays, Sharon Latta, Jackie McAtee, Kathleen Murphy, Anick Neider, Tish Osborn, Carol Robson, Elise Smith, and Candy Woodson.

The support and encouragement provided by Candy Woodson, president of the Feingold Association of the United States, have aided greatly in the development of this book. Her extensive experience with hyperactive children and their families has made her aware of the need for a book such as this one, and she has facilitated its creation in many ways.

Sharon Latta, president of the Feingold Association of the Northwest, has given much time and energy toward the development of this book and encouragement in its writing.

The Salem Oregon Family YMCA encouraged the offering of parent education courses for parents of hyperactive children for several years immediately prior to the publication of this book. My experience in conducting these courses provided much of the information that appears in this work.

Academic and school issues were helpfully expanded by the contributions of Jane Hanrahan, Ethel Jones, JoAnne Perrington, and Doris Woodfield. The combined experience of these persons is impressive, and their suggestions for improving the book helped greatly, especially for the chapters dealing with school adjustment.

Medical and mental health professionals whose opinions I respect greatly reviewed portions of the manuscript and offered helpful suggestions. These persons include Maurice Bullard, Dr. Paul Fine, Dr. Ray Lowe, Floy Pepper, Dr. John Platt, Dr. David Sessions, Dr. John Schulte, Dr. Steve Swenson, and Dr. Grant Thorsett.

Don Cowles, pharmacist and learning disabilities specialtist, provided much helpful information on the Feingold nutritional program and on additive-free medicines for hyperactive children.

Dr. Clement Vickery shared his keen understanding of hyperactive children through our many years of professional work together. Dr. Vickery, along with Don Derby, developed an early form of the hyperactivity screening checklist. Although I am responsible for the subsequent refinement of the checklist and the research on its effectiveness, credit must go to Dr. Vickery for his role in inspiring me to pursue the project.

My dear wife, Linda, and my delightful children deserve final mention, because their sacrifice was the greatest. For their patience and love I am indebted to them beyond expression, and my love for them is also without measure.

Foreword

Parenting is hard work. Being the parent of a hyperactive child is even harder work. It is a very emotional experience. Many of the emotions are positive: warmth, excitement, wonder, satisfaction, and hope. But many are negative: frustration, disappointment, guilt, fear, anger, despair, and confusion. Being the parent of a hyperactive child is demanding and challenging and requires considerable time, patience, and understanding. The time and energy required can impose stresses on the marital relationship and the family. Patience can wear thin and undermine family harmony. Lack of understanding and confusion about how to raise the child can undo the very best parenting efforts.

Dr. Taylor's book enables parents to gain a better understanding of the child's uniqueness and his impact on the family. It also provides them with a wealth of information and practical suggestions for effectively dealing with the hyperactive child in the family, in the neighborhood, and at school. My experience has shown that while parents of hyperactive children have the strength and energy and do take the extra time required to attend to those children's needs, many lack the understanding and information necessary to effectively meet the demands and stresses of having a hyperactive child in the family.

Dr. Taylor's book reflects his intense involvement with parents of hyperactive children, directly addresses concerns that parents have, and answers the questions that they most want answered. As a first step toward helping their child, parents need to understand their own feelings toward the child, and they must deal with those feelings. Dr. Taylor provides useful suggestions to cope with this problem. But this topic is only one of many covered in the outstanding chapters of his book. Also included are explanations of the three most popular treatment methods—counseling, medication, and nutrition management. The advantages and disadvantages associated with each are discussed in detail. All parents are concerned about their hyperactive child's self-esteem, and suggestions are offered for strengthening his sense of self-worth. Unique to Dr. Taylor's book is the recognition of the emotional stresses experienced by parents in response to the hyperactive child.

Probably no other term has stirred up as much controversy and confusion as the term "hyperactivity." Confusion exists regarding how to define and diagnose hyperactivity, and what constitutes its appropriate treatment and management. This confusion is magnified by lack of agreement among physicians, mental health workers, and school personnel. Really understanding the hyperactive child can bring about the "potential positive effects" described by Dr. Taylor. Understanding, as I use the term, means both empathic understanding and "to know thoroughly." Empathic understanding involves the sensitivity to be able to see the child's world through the child's eyes, enabling the parent to understand how the hyperactive child feels and how the world affects him. Knowing thoroughly includes knowing yourself—the strengths and resources that you have as a parent, your marital relationship, how to complement your partner, the dynamics of your family and how your child affects those dynamics, what form of treatment works best for your child, sound child-rearing practices, and how to assist in the personal, social, and educational growth of your child.

In this book parents are given suggestions for resolving their own emotional conflicts, stresses arising from strained parent-child relationships. Destructive patterns in the marital relationship are discussed, and solutions are given for correcting those patterns. The nature of difficulties with peers and siblings is explained, and specific methods are outlined for improving those relationships.

An Adlerian approach to discipline is portrayed in detail. This feature provides a refreshing new look at disciplining the hyperactive child, because "behavioral management" techniques have received the most attention in the literature on this area. Dr. Taylor's book also includes ideas on organizing recreation and play, and on rebuilding family harmony.

Not only is parenting a hyperactive child hard work, but teaching him is also hard work. Dr. Taylor's book includes excellent classroom teaching strategies and provides suggestions for getting the most out of school personnel.

I have been interested in the special needs of hyperactive children for almost a decade. I have listened to the concerns of overwhelmed parents, frustrated teachers, and unhappy and defeated children. I have supported parents and teachers and have assisted them in developing programs for meeting the special needs of the hyperactive child. I have nurtured the bruised and fragile self-esteems of these children.

I wish Dr. Taylor's book could have been available ten years ago, but I am happy a book of this quality is available now. Parents and others interested in hyperactive children will find *The Hyperactive Child and the Family: The Complete What-To-Do Handbook* an excellent resource.

THOMAS N. FAIRCHILD, PH.D.

Chairman, Guidance and Counseling Dept., University of Idaho, and author of *Managing the Hyperactive Child in the Classroom*

Introduction

Hyperactivity is a challenge, and like any challenge it can be both a blessing and a curse.

Any parent of a hyperactive child can tell horror stories based on personal experience. From the hyperactive fetus who bruises his pregnant mother's ribs to the seven-year-old who takes a bicycle apart without the aid of tools, there are dozens of stressful, difficult aspects to family life with a hyperactive child.

Ideally the experience of raising a hyperactive child will strengthen the parents. It will stimulate them to put great effort and concentration into their relationship with each other and into their roles as their child's guides. In their hunt for resources with which to counter the destructive effects of the hyperactivity, they can stretch and grow as individuals. Where there is struggle, there can be growth. Much can be done, and the sooner the better.

Potential Positive Effects

The experience of raising a hyperactive child can help parents gain a sense of community with others. They may stop being judgmental toward other parents, particularly those who have difficulties with their own children. They may become more willing to accept help from others. At the same time, they may learn to recognize and accept the errors, gaps in knowledge, and shortcomings of professional helpers. In short, they may become aware of the basic humanity and equality of people, regardless of their social station or number of graduate degrees.

Bringing up a hyperactive child will either enhance or injure the parents' relationships with each other; its effect will not be neutral. They will either rise to the occasion and become closer, or they will crumble under the stress and become more emotionally distant from each other. They might come to see the necessity for a weekly date and for frequent weekends away together in order to strengthen their strained relations. They may search out sources of renewal in the form of marriage enrichment programs. By taking steps such as these, they can achieve a deeper commitment to their relationship than do many other couples.

As the marriage of the parents goes, so goes the family. The entire family will either become more united or more divided in response to the common enemy of hyperactivity. The hyperactive child can help create and be a part of that unity. Everyone in the family can share a sense of mission and purpose, a common goal of working to counter a shared stress which exists through no fault of any one family member. For example, the family might join the hyperactive child on the Feingold nutritional program. Parents can become creative in their search for things to do together as a family, and in doing so they will be giving devotion and strength that surpasses that of many other families.

Dealing with the hyperactivity can help parents develop their skills and knowledge about child rearing. They can learn how to: make joint decisions on a cooperative basis with regard to the children; become skilled at structuring their home to prevent misbehavior; find meaningful routines that contribute to a quiet orderliness in the household; apply the family-council method for keeping communication open. They can attend parent education classes and discussion groups in order to improve their ability to make wise leadership decisions. In these and other ways, they can be stimulated to become more knowledgeable and more effective than the average parent.

Approaches to Hyperactivity

There is a great deal of disagreement over the definition of hyperactivity. Some medical and mental health professionals diagnose too many children as hyperactive, seeing it when it is not actually present. Others diagnose it too infrequently, failing to recognize it when it occurs. Estimates of its frequency of occurrence vary widely, ranging from about 3 to about 20 percent of all children. It is safe to conclude that there is at least one hyperactive child in every average school classroom and at least one hyperactive child in every ten families. Most of these children continue to show signs of hyperactivity throughout adolescence and into adulthood. Hyperactivity appears to have increased during the last two decades. There is no agreement as to why this increase has occurred, but many claim that it is in part because of the more than five thousand additives used in foods during these twenty years.

Just as there is disagreement about who is and who is not hyperactive, there is no unity of opinion about how to treat it. When all is said and done, the final choice of method of treatment, or combination of methods, must be an individual decision, based on the parents' awareness of the family's needs and capabilities. This book discusses and evaluates the three most common treatment approaches: treatment by the Feingold nutritional program; treatment by medication; and treatment by professional counseling. After studying the available options, the parents must make the final choice.

How to Use This Book

The focus throughout this book is on strengthening and rebuilding the feelings of self-worth within each member of the family, as well as strengthening the love bonds among family members.

This focus on family relationships, including the child's effect on the parents' marriage, the child at play, and rebuilding family harmony, is intended to provide answers to the hardest questions that are faced by parents of the hyperactive child. These are vital issues which receive little or no mention in other books on the hyperactive child.

Many of the principles of family living given in this book stem from the pioneering work of Alfred Adler, an Austrian psychiatrist who developed many important concepts during the first half of this century.

Adler recognized the enormous potential that each individual has for making choices from personal strength while almost all leaders in his field were concluding that people were helplessly buffeted by instincts. Much of the material in this book on sibling relationships, feelings of personal inferiority, the effects of each child's perceived position in the family, encouragement for strengthening self-esteem, and order and discipline within the family must be credited ultimately to Adler and his student, Dr. Rudolph Dreikurs.

Though addressed primarily to parents, this book should be read by anyone who wants to learn more about hyperactivity. Parents may want to give the book to relatives, child care personnel, physicians, mental health counselors, teachers, or others who assist them in managing their child.

This book can be used as source material for a discussion group comprised of parents of hyperactive children. Such a group can pool knowledge, experiences, and approaches to hyperactivity for everyone's benefit. Two chapters could be discussed at each meeting so that the entire book would be covered in just a few weeks. Discussion questions for each chapter are provided in the Appendices section. A discussion group does not require a professional leader.

The information presented in *The Hyperactive Child and the Family* was gathered largely from my personal experiences with several hundred parents of hyperactive, learning-disabled children, as well as from the children themselves. My background in parent education and family counseling enabled me to translate those experiences into what I hope will be practical help for parents, to help them understand the hyperactive child and the family and to make life easier and happier for everyone concerned.

                                                  JOHN F. TAYLOR, PH.D.
Salem, Oregon
June 1980

THE
HYPERACTIVE CHILD
AND THE FAMILY

THE TRAIT OF HYPERACTIVITY

Hyperactivity is difficult to define. There is little agreement among mental health, academic, and medical professionals as to its exact diagnosis, causes, and best approaches to treatment. Because of this lack of clear understanding of hyperactivity by those who are involved with it, parents will no doubt receive conflicting opinions from professional helpers in various fields.

Hyperactivity is an inclusive label for a large cluster of traits that are described in this section. Children who are not hyperactive may show a few of these traits. A child can be said to be exhibiting increasingly severe hyperactivity to the extent that more and more of these traits are present.

As a further aid to identifying true hyperactivity, the Taylor Hyperactivity Screening Checklist is also presented in this section. See the Appendices section for a description of the research background of this easy-to-use checklist.

Chapter 1

Is Your Child Hyperactive?

From the time that they first sense that something is different about their child, the parents of a hyperactive child face question upon question and stress upon stress. Answers don't come—just more questions and more frustrations. They are told that the child is merely "going through a phase," that he will "grow out of it," or that "boys will be boys." When these casual dismissals of the child's problem prove inaccurate; the parents are told that the child is mentally ill, mentally retarded, a slow learner, or handicapped in a vague and undefined way. Then the parents become terror-stricken and even more confused. As time goes on, they learn to rely more on their own intuition and experience than on anything else in raising the child because other sources of information and guidance are misleading and inconsistent.

Hyperactivity Is a Symptom

There are a number of causes for temporary nervousness and increased activity in children. Diseases such as diabetes, hypoglycemia, and allergies can produce hyperactive states. Hyperactivity can also appear as a symptom in some types of extreme emotional disturbance. It can be the result of severe physical damage to brain matter, such as a skull fracture. The child who is nervous because of conflict and stress in the home may become temporarily hyperactive.

The majority of children who are hyperactive show some of these symptoms *consistently*, day in and day out. There may be dramatic switches in the child's behavior as he goes from situation to situation, but he will be *consistently* fidgety in school or *consistently* pushy at home. The types, the number, the severity of the symptoms vary, so that each hyperactive child shows a unique pattern of behavior and personality. There are, however, certain similarities among hyperactive children.

The child in whom hyperactivity is a consistent symptom is usually diagnosed medically as showing a hyperkinetic reaction, or an attentional deficit disorder. First-born children are more often hyperactive than later-born children. According to estimates four out of five hyperactive children are boys. The apparently higher incidence among boys than among girls is a common occurrence for many diseases and handicaps, and it is generally thought to result from genetic factors. Also, there may be some tendency among teachers and parents to notice hyperactive boys more quickly than they notice hyperactive girls. Hyperactive girls sometimes are excused as being simply tomboyish, while hyperactive boys quickly become obvious because of their high degree of activity and rowdiness.

Hyperactivity Is Part of the Learning-Disabilities Syndrome

Some diseases known to cause gross damage to brain cells, such as encephalitis, have been found also to produce hyperactivity as a symptom. In the 1950s the term "minimal brain damage" was developed to describe the assumed cause of certain behavior changes and learning problems of children. These children showed behavior similar to that of children with known brain damage—hyperactivity, impulsiveness, perceptual problems, and a host of related symptoms. In most cases, however, medical tests did not show any physical damage to the brains of these children. The term was later changed to "minimal brain dysfunction" to indicate malfunctioning of the brain cells without apparent physical damage to them.

The collection of symptoms eventually came to be called "learning disabilities," and various refinements in the definition have been tried. It has been estimated that less than half of all children with learning disabilities are recognized and that only a fraction receive adequate help in schools.

Characteristics of the Hyperactive Child

The traits listed in this chapter are the symptoms most often found among children who can be classified as showing a hyperkinetic reaction or attentional deficit disorder. Taken together, these twenty traits comprise the learning disabilities syndrome. For ease of reading, the list is divided into three categories: mental difficulties, physical difficulties, and emotional difficulties. Not all hyperactive children have all of these symptoms, but most hyperactive children have most of them. Although many of these traits appear in the majority of children from time to time, they indicate hyperactivity when the child is unable to change them and when they appear consistently.

Mental Difficulties

• DISTRACTIBILITY. As you read this paragraph, you are focusing your attention on this page and are to some extent blocking out the other messages received by your brain. Your brain is preventing the majority of information that it is receiving from coming into your awareness, so that you can be free to concentrate on this collection of words. While you read, your ears are sending messages, telling your brain what they hear, regardless of whether you have been aware of hearing anything. Your taste buds are sending messages about the tastes that are now present in your mouth, regardless of whether you have been aware of tasting anything. The nerve endings in your nose are sending messages about the odors in the air that you are breathing at this moment, regardless of whether you have been aware of smelling anything. In addition, many messages have been coming to your brain from inside your body, informing it of such things as your degree of hunger, the sense of pressure that you feel from your clothing, the temperature and humidity of the air that is in contact with your skin, the exact location and condition of every body part, and thousands of other bits of information.

How have you been able to block out that flood of information in order to focus on these words? You have a "gatekeeper" that allows only relevant, useful, important information into your conscious awareness. Your gatekeeper makes it possible for you to pay attention to one thing while ignoring thousands of other messages that your brain is receiving at the same moment.

The hyperactive child has a faulty gatekeeper. He has little ability to block out noises in order to concentrate. The noise outside the window is just as important as the arithmetic problem that he is supposed to be copying from the blackboard. The noise made by a dropped pencil is just as important as the words the teacher is saying. Experiencing the feel of the cloth rubbing against skin, created by wiggling in the chair, is just as important as answering the next question in the test at school.

The child may appear to be working at school, but the teacher may find that the work is not completed. The child may be distracted by such incidental things as stray marks or scratches in books and papers that others would not even notice. To the hyperactive child, however, they are just as commanding of attention as the words that are printed on those pages.

When the child is looking at his mother, he might be paying more attention to the noises in the house than to what she is telling him at the moment. The pattern of the colors on the wall is just as important as the memory of the errand that the parent has just asked the child to do. The sensations of body movement are just as important as the threat of punishment if the child doesn't sit still at the dinner table.

The hyperactive child is poor at focusing concentration, channeling effort, and saving energy for useful purposes. It is as if he is drawn by an automatic reflex to pay attention to any noise, any stray flash of light, any sounds made by others, or any internal body state. The result is a very short attention span and a tendency to be easily distracted from what is important by what is unimportant. Hyperactive children often seem to have their antennae up at all times; they seem to be aware of everything that is going on around them.

• MENTAL CONFUSION. The hyperactive child usually has trouble recognizing a figure that stands out from the background. Instead, he may see figure and background as if they are equally prominent and intermingled. This trait also applies to the child's handling of ideas. Decisions are difficult to make, and establishing priorities is seldom done. The child may have trouble remembering what is important. He may put just as much effort into remembering unimportant facts and lessons as he puts into the important things that he is supposed to be learning.

There is usually confusion about instructions and directions. The child may be unable to follow directions without prompting and additional help. When asked to do two or three things, he may remember to do only the first one. Directions that are given verbally are especially difficult for the child to remember and to make priorities for.

The hyperactive child usually has trouble organizing and arranging his schoolwork. He may gain a reputation for being scatterbrained and careless at school. He may start new projects without finishing them.

The child's performance may vary greatly from day to day. A skill or new bit of knowledge may seem to be mastered but then be forgotten a few hours later, or he may remember it for several consecutive days, and then suddenly forget it.

• CONCRETE THINKING. Read this sentence: "Certain four-wheeled vehicles, of which the average United States family has more than one, require a fuel which is sold from pumps in places called stations and which is refined from crude oil."

Now re-read it at least once, with the goal of being able to summarize it by expressing its basic idea in three to five words.

This long sentence can easily be shortened into statements such as, "cars need gas" or "cars get gas from stations." In shortening the sentence, word substitution is necessary. Nowhere in that sentence do the words "cars," "need," "get," or "gas" appear. In finding new words or in rearranging words to shorten the sentence, the ability to organize thoughts and words is necessary. This is concept formation, or abstract reasoning ability, a skill that the hyperactive child lacks. The thinking of the hyperactive child is, instead, concrete and literal.

The child may act as if his mind were much like a tape recorder, being able to remember only word-for-word messages. There is little ability to process or reorganize the messages into any sort of sequence or priority. In trying to summarize the above sentence, the child might say: "Certain four-wheeled vehicles . . . family . . . fuel . . . stations . . . oil."

Because of thinking only literally, the child may have difficulty understanding the content of what he reads. The abstract reasoning that is part of arithmetic may also be very difficult for the child.

The child may have trouble thinking hypothetically, in a "what if" fashion. Rather than using an example as a basis for a general guideline, the child is likely either to personalize it or to misinterpret it. After hearing the fable of the fox and the grapes, which involves the fox's rationalizing that he did not want the grapes after he found it impossible to reach them, the child might get sidetracked into a discussion of grapes or foxes, or he might point out that foxes can't talk. He may be unable to understand the abstract principle or teaching point in the fable. After hearing about the method used by two other children to settle an argument, he may not be able to apply it to his own life because the fight did not directly involve him.

The child may have trouble learning indirectly or applying information from previous experiences to current ones. He may claim not to know a fact in geography because he has never been there. He may not know how to do something that he has seen others do because he has never previously done it. He may not understand the meaning of a statement because he has never heard it before. When asked to use common sense in a new situation, he may appear lost and aimless. The hyperactive child seems to need routine, habit, or close and direct supervision in order to deal with new or ambiguous situations.

The hyperactive child usually has a great deal of trouble connecting cause and effect. It is difficult to teach the child that the cat won't be friendly if teased, that other children won't play if bullied, that pets will get sick if not fed and watered, and that low grades will be the result of poor effort at school.

• RIGID ACTIONS. The hyperactive child lacks flexibility, tending to be rigid in his approach to others and to new situations. He may have trouble switching from one phase or type of activity to another. The child may be unable to free himself from useless actions, even when those actions are obviously no longer helpful. At school he may give the same answer to several questions in a row. If he has already drawn a circle, he may continue to draw circles even when asked to copy a square. The child will persist in his original approach longer than other children will, and he will hesitate to reject his poor solution even after many unsuccessful experiences.

There is poor adjustment to environmental change. Rearranging the furniture in the living room can upset the child, as can the arrival of house guests or any last-minute change in family plans.

• DIFFICULTY IN EXPRESSING FEELINGS WITH WORDS. The child may not be able to find the words to express emotions which are obviously present. Instead of describing the feelings, the child is more likely to bottle them up, then discharge them in an emotional explosion. Stuttering and stammering can sometimes result from this inability to deal with emotion through language.

• AIMLESSNESS. The hyperactive child usually appears to be inconsistent, so that parents feel off balance, as if the child is always one step ahead of them and they never know what he is going to do next. The child often gains a reputation for being unpredictable.

The life of the child usually has a disjointed, episodic nature. There seems to be no flow, no accommodation to change or to the needs of others. It may seem that he is not able to profit from past errors and move forward in life. The child's life may seem barren and without direction.

There may be little foresight, planning, or thoughtfulness. The child may generally tend to do things without considering the possible consequences.

• PERCEPTUAL DIFFICULTIES. The child may show confusion about common opposites. Differentiating items that are upside-down or inside-out may be difficult. The child might, for example, put on clothing or stockings inside-out without realizing it. Reversals may take place in reading and writing. Letters like d and b, w and m, and p and q may be used incorrectly in place of each other. Sometimes the reversals take the form of exchanging the positions of letters within a word, as when dog is read or spelled as god, was is read or spelled as saw, or is is read or spelled as si.

There may be various problems with spatial relationships. The child may have trouble telling the difference between an object that is vertical and one that is horizontal. The child may have difficulty recognizing relationships like over, under, beside, and between. Such skills as reading maps, telling time, and doing arithmetic problems require high spatial relationship awareness that is often beyond the ability of the child. The child often is not able to perceive and understand clearly the relative positions of the numbers and letters.

Right-left discrimination, which is a combination of spatial relationships and opposition, may be difficult for the hyperactive child. He might put shoes on the wrong feet or may have trouble remembering which hand is left and which is right.

Visual perceptual problems include difficulty with seeing things as a whole. Instead, a picture or design is broken down in the child's mind into two or three separate parts which are not a unified whole. Reading may plod along, so that the child reads only one word at a time with no flow from one word to the next.

A similar problem occurs because the child may be unable to fill in parts that are missing in what he sees or hears. For example, he may have difficulty remembering what comes next in a song that he has been taught many times, or he may not be able to fill in the correct numbers in the middle of a sequence of numbers, even if he has been given the beginning and ending of the sequence.

Visual perceptual problems can be especially handicapping when the child is writing and drawing. Printing may appear sloppy. Handwriting may show a varying slant from letter to letter. The child's artistic ability may be poor. He may be literally unable to write or draw what he sees. He may see a five-pointed star, for example, but be able to draw only a four-pointed one. He may see a slanted parallelogram but be able to draw only a square. Even the left-to-right movement of the child's eyes during reading may be difficult. There is the possibility of his occasionally trying to read from right to left.

There may be poor depth perception, resulting in clumsiness and awkwardness. The child may perceive corners of objects as protruding farther than they do, thinking that things are sticking out toward him when they actually are not.

Various perceptual problems can also affect the child's skill in using his sense of hearing. There may be problems in hearing the separate sounds made by the various letters. The child may accidentally omit letters or words when reading. There may be poor perception of rhyme. Analyzing words into sound units may be troublesome; "ing" may be pronounced by the child as "in" and "g." The child's ability to hear melody, harmony, or rhythm in music may be impaired, and the child may have difficulty singing on key.

Perception of his own internal states may be incorrect. He may think that his bladder is full when it is not. He may not feel hunger even though he has not eaten for a long time. He may not feel pain to a normal degree. It is not uncommon for hyperactive children to injure themselves severely and fail to report the injury until much later. There may be daytime wetting and soiling because the child is unaware of bowel and bladder activity.

● POOR AWARENESS OF BODY POSITION. The child may not have a clear understanding of his body position in relation to his surroundings. He may bump into or stumble over things, and he may be generally clumsy. Accidentally knocking objects off of tables is a common occurrence. The child may easily become lost and disoriented in new settings or in office buildings. He may be unable to maintain a sense of direction and may complain of becoming turned around or disoriented easily when in unfamiliar places Some of the child's destructiveness stems from this symptom

Physical Difficulties

• CONSTANT MOVEMENT. This trait is one of the two that form hyperactivity in its narrowest sense. Many hyperactive children were unusually active before they were born. Occasionally mothers report bruised ribs or other internal damage from a hyperactive fetus. The hyperactive child acts as if he is being driven by a giant mainspring that is wound too tightly.

During infancy, the child may rock his crib excessively and in other ways be unusually active. As the child grows older, there may be a tendency to run and jump rather than walk, even when walking is asked for by supervising adults.

The child may show poor channeling of energy, with irrelevant and useless movements of various body parts. He may act jumpy and fidgety, with some body part always rocking, wiggling, or moving.

The child may need to be doing something all the time and be unable simply to sit quietly and restfully. Even when his attention is on the television set, the child may change body position, make tapping noises, or have some sort of constant movement. It may be difficult for the child to sit quietly through a meal without getting up. The child may grimace frequently or have a tic.

At school the child may receive frequent reminders to sit down, turn around, leave nearby children and objects alone, and tend to schoolwork. He may tend to poke, touch, feel, and grab; keeping his hands out of mischief may seem difficult or impossible. For example, he may compulsively touch everything in stores, and he may touch other children, lockers, and hallway walls when walking through school.

The child may be consistently noisy, making lots of clicks, whistles, and other sounds with mouth and body, and getting a reputation for being a chatterbox and having a very loud voice.

• VARIATIONS IN DEVELOPMENTAL RATES. Some hyperactive children develop abilities very rapidly. A hyperactive child may walk and talk earlier in life than most other infants. Sometimes they skip some stages altogether: for example, learning to walk without first learning to crawl.

More often the hyperactive child will have the opposite characteristics—a slowness in passing the milestones of infancy and early childhood. Some hyperactive children don't start crawling until after ten months and don't start walking until after eighteen months. Some show delayed development of speech and a small vocabulary.

• PHYSICAL ABNORMALITIES. Seizures, allergies, and a sweet tooth may occur. There may be a craving for cakes and pastries, candy, jelly, and sugar. The most common allergic reactions among hyperactive children occur with chocolate, corn and corn products, eggs, milk, nuts, pork, sugar, and wheat products.

Some of the child's reflexes may not function normally. When asked to produce a rapid back and forth movement with one hand, the child may automatically produce an identical movement in the other hand without realizing it. There may be left or mixed dominance; that is, the favored eye, hand, and foot might not all be on the right side.

Various visual difficulties can occur among hyperactive children. The eyes may be physically abnormal. They might not maintain a steady gaze but instead may roam and look away when the child is asked to look at something.

Incidental aspects of the placement of the eyes and ears on the head, the structure of the mouth, the size and spacing of fingers and toes, and other minor characteristics have been found to occur in abnormal manifestations among hyperactive boys. These minor traits, in and of themselves, cause no problem in the life of the hyperactive child. It is also interesting to note that the combination of blue eyes and blond hair, both recessive traits, occurs about twice as often among hyperactive children as among non-hyperactive children.

• NERVOUSNESS COMPULSIONS. The child may seem driven to repeat certain behaviors which are commonly considered to indicate nervousness. There may be thumb sucking, nail biting, scratching and picking at sores and fingernails, teeth grinding, and head banging. These actions may stem from a number of causes but often do not indicate nervousness in the ordinary sense. For example, many hyperactive children complain of itching a lot, and they scratch themselves a great deal in response to the tingling, itching sensation they feel on their skin.

• UNUSUAL SLEEP. The hyperactive child may not want to sleep and may oppose going to bed, even though he has been quite active throughout the day. It may be hard for parents to get the child to go to sleep after he is in bed.

Some hyperactive children have very shallow sleep, which may occur in short periods rather than in the standard eight- to ten-hour period. The child's sleeping pattern may be irregular. The sleep may be restless, with excessive body movement during the sleep.

In contrast to the shallow, restless sleep of some hyperactive children, others have an extremely deep sleep, with nightmares, sleep talking, sleep walking, or bed wetting.

• COORDINATION DIFFICULTIES. The hyperactive child may have a poor sense of balance. Riding a bicycle, a two-wheeled scooter, or a skateboard may be difficult. The trampoline is a particularly telltale device; the hyperactive child with a coordination symptom will find it a very difficult piece of gymnastic equipment to use.

There may be general awkwardness of movement and a clumsy gait. The child may find it difficult to hop on one foot, to jump rope, or to skip, and may be poor at ball sports.

The hyperactive child may be unable to place his hands in particular positions, especially with his eyes closed. Rapid back and forth movements of fingers, as in finger tapping, may be difficult. He also may have more difficulty than other children of the same age in learning how to color within the lines and how to manipulate buttons and shoelaces.

• SENSITIVITY REACTIONS. The child may show a dramatic increase in hyperactivity when exposed to any of several irritants through skin contact, inhalation, or eating or drinking. Common offenders include artificially flavored and colored food, perfumed toiletries, fumes of petroleum products and cleaning agents, TRIS flame retardant in clothes, some commercial modeling compounds, bubble bath, chemically treated paper like that used in clothes dryers, and food containing chemical preservatives. (See Table 2 in Chapter 3.)

Emotional Difficulties

• SELF-CENTEREDNESS. The hyperactive child usually seems to have little awareness of his impact on others. Social judgment and self-analysis are foreign to him. He may do hurtful things without meaning to hurt others, then may act surprised when others show anger. The child may expect others not to be displeased when he misbehaves. The child's voice is apt to be too loud for whatever situation he is in.

The child may blame others and external circumstances for his difficulties rather than accept his own responsibility for contributing to those difficulties. The problem is usually seen as someone else's fault. The child has great difficulty thinking of any need for self-improvement; he seldom admits to a personal weakness or self-defeating trait.

The child's own wants, needs, and whims often appear to be his dominant and primary concern. The child may be bullheaded and stubborn about getting his own way. He may be inflexible and may refuse to negotiate or even to hear others' points of view. When denied, the child may pester and harp on the issue until the parent, teacher, or other person gives in.

Falling into line with others' needs and wants may be unpleasant for the child; he may want the rules changed or demand to be the exception. On the other hand, the child may be zealous in enforcing a rule that is to his advantage. The child may pretend to have an "I don't care" attitude if threatened or punished by parents or teachers.

• IMPATIENCE. The child is typically negativistic, contrary, and hard to please. Parents may sense that the child is always complaining and displeased about something. The child may be impulsive and do things without first asking permission. The impatience may show up in the child's behavior when he stands in line: he may poke, push, and shove to get ahead, or, better yet, be first. The hyperactive child seems unable to wait for anything!

• RECKLESSNESS. The child may not be diligent. He may make lots of careless errors and take a slipshod approach to tasks. The child may be lighthearted and carefree, as though he takes nothing seriously.

Acts may be committed which indicate a disregard for safety and health, with no awareness of obvious dangers and risks. A devil-may-care approach may characterize the child, who may seem to have no fear of heights, strangers, animals, traffic, traveling alone for great distances, or wandering away from home.

The child may be irresponsible in play, being too rough with toys, objects, furniture, and pets. The child may be destructive and may set fires.

Social inhibitions may be rare. The typical hyperactive child is assertive, intrusive, and without shyness. Curiosity may seem unbridled; the child may be too curious and too nosey.

• EXTREME EMOTIONS. There is usually a lack of restraint or cushioning of the child's emotions which are often expressed in raw, overwhelming and extreme form. The child may seem to be ruled by emotion, with rapid mood changes in which his personality seems to alter drastically. The child may be excitable and quick to react emotionally to any event.

There is often a low frustration tolerance. The child is likely to be irritable and unable to accept no for an answer from parents or teachers. Anger might be expressed by vicious and extreme acts and tantrums. Outbursts of temper may be frequent and violent, and the child may seem to be out of control. Minor frustrations may trigger a major tantrum. If the child is spanked, he may fly apart emotionally, and the situation may be worsened rather than improved.

• CONSCIENCE GAPS. The child may not be able to keep friends, though at first there may be no difficulty in attracting them. There may be fighting with other children as the friendships deteriorate. The child may try to manipulate other children into various alliances. He may eventually be rejected and disliked by the majority of the children at school and in the neighborhood.

The hyperactive child often takes on an aggressive role in relation to other children. He may bully and start fights, harass other children physically, or he may needle them with cutting words, especially when the other children are in a weak or defenseless position. The hyperactive child may be cruel to animals in general but may make an exception of his own pet.

He may interrupt others' conversations and be rude, tactless, and overbearing. He may invade the bedrooms of siblings, violate their privacy, and use their belongings without permission. Shoplifting and other forms of stealing are a possibility.

Attracted to the misbehavior of others, the child may be generally disobedient, undisciplined, and uncontrollable. When caught, he may lie and become defiant. When punished, he is unlikely to learn from the experience, other than to avoid being caught in the future.

Hyperactivity during Adolescence and Adulthood

At puberty, the total amount of hyperactivity may seem to decrease in hyperactive children. Many explanations have been offered for this interesting apparent change. Although there is no general agreement about which, if any, is the best explanation, these are the three most widely held:

• BRAIN GROWTH FULFILLMENT. Some theorists have suggested that hyperactivity might be caused by the fact that different parts of the brain grow and mature at different rates. The cerebrum, which is the "brake pedal" of the mind, may not mature at a rate sufficient to counterbalance the other parts of the brain, with the result that the child shows deficiencies in cerebral functioning. At puberty, or shortly thereafter, the brain is known to reach its final and full growth, its adult size. One result might be that the slower maturing parts of the brain have caught up with the faster maturing parts, so that all parts of the brain cross the finish line together. The brain is then in balance, and the biochemical imbalances causing hyperactivity disappear.

• HORMONAL CHANGES. The vast chemical changes of puberty, which affect many body parts and systems, may also affect brain chemistry in such a way as to create a new form of chemical balance.

• INCREASED SELF-CONTROL AND SOCIAL AWARENESS. The adolescent has increased concern about how he appears to others. He is more willing and more able to control behavior in accordance with group pressure and group norms. The adolescent has a desire to avoid doing things that would bring rejection or embarrassment at the hands of the all-important peer group. The adolescent's concern for meshing in with the group may allow him to exert a new measure of self-control on impulsiveness and foolish recklessness, which may no longer serve any useful purpose.

Many hyperactive children do not show an apparent decrease in hyperactivity during adolescence. For these persons, the stresses relating to self-esteem, peer relationships, family, and school multiply and magnify each other, often propelling the child down a self-destructive path. Many untreated hyperactive adolescents find their way into the juvenile and, eventually, the adult penal systems.

The children who do not decrease in apparent hyperactivity during adolescence may continue being hyperactive in their adult years. Many of them are able to adapt to life with reasonable success, though still showing some telltale signs: talkativeness, constant movement, starting many new projects but not completing them, being too intrusive and tactless in social gatherings, or similar traits. Some, however, continue in an aimless way, blaming others for their difficulties and developing addictive habits to alcohol or drugs.

Hyperactivity is apparently a lifelong disorder. Although it may appear to lessen, it probably does not disappear. While no longer crippled by the hyperactivity, those who have shown an apparent decrease during adolescence still have a psychological limp during their adult years.

A Screening Checklist for Hyperactivity

There has been a definite and important need for a quick screening test which a parent, teacher, counselor, physician, or other concerned adult can use to determine whether or not a child is indeed hyperactive. The Taylor Hyperactivity Screening Checklist has been developed for that purpose.

This checklist contains twenty-one of the most consistent traits among hyperactive children. The opposites of these twenty-one traits are also rare among hyperactive children. Children who have most of these traits are hyperactive, while those who do not are not hyperactive.

This checklist makes the first crude division between hyperkinetic reaction and anything else. It is *not* a final proof of any diagnosis or condition. It is not a comprehensive list of all symptoms often shown by hyperactive children. Instead it lists the most *differentiating* symptoms, those which are very likely to occur exclusively in hyperactive children. Diagnosis of hyperactivity and its underlying causes goes far beyond the scope of this checklist.

TABLE 1   The Taylor Hyperactivity Screening Checklist

For each of the twenty-one behaviors, put an X in one of the three boxes to show what is typical for the child. Rate the child's behavior when the child is *not* being supervised, helped, or reminded; when the child is *not* receiving medication or nutrition management to control hyperactivity; when the child is *not* watching television. Indicate the trend—which direction the child's behavior is leaning.

Compared with other children of the same age, this child shows behavior:

Activity	A. More like this	B. In between or don't know	C. More like this	Activity
1. Quiet when sitting				Noisy and talkative when sitting
2. Voice volume is soft or average				Voice is generally too loud
3. Few mouth or body noises				Makes lots of clicks, whistles, and sounds with mouth or body
4. Walks at appropriate times				Runs and jumps rather than walks
5. Keeps hands to self				Pokes, touches, feels, and grabs
6. Appears calm, can be still				Always has something moving; fidgets with hands or feet; jumpy
7. Can just sit				Has to be doing something when sitting, to occupy self
8. Concentrates and blocks out distractions				Gets distracted by noises, people, etc.
9. Slow to react, thinks before acting				Quick to react, reacts on impulse

Activity	A. More like this	B. In between or don't know	C. More like this	Activity
10. Finishes one thing before starting another				Starts many new things without finishing any
11. Obeys directions and follows orders				Disobeys and needs supervision or reminding
12. Avoids joining into others' mischief				Attracted by and gets drawn into others' mischief
13. Understands why others are displeased after misbehavior				Expects others not to be displeased by misbehavior, or does not realize that misbehavior has occurred
14. Thinks ahead to later consequences				Does things without considering consequences, doesn't plan ahead
15. Cooperates, obeys and enforces rules				Wants rules changed, wants to be the exception
16. Concerned about punishments and consequences				Pretends to have an "I don't care" attitude if threatened or punished
17. Constant mood with mild or slow mood changes; calm				Rapid and extreme mood changes, happy one minute and hostile the next; moody
18. Gives up when denied by parent or teacher				When denied, child pesters, harps on it, doesn't give up

Activity	A. More like this	B. In be- tween or don't know	C. More like this	Activity
19. Easy going, can accept frustration, can take no for an answer				Irritable, can't accept frustration, can't take no for an an- swer
20. Doesn't try to bother or hurt others with words				Needles, teases, picks on others with words
21. Emotions don't dis- rupt relationships, are reasonably re- strained				Emotions are ex- treme rather than moderated; child seems ruled by them; very hostile or very affectionate

The score is the total number of items in Column B plus *twice* the number of items rated in Column C. The range of possible scores is 0 to 42. The lowest possible score would be obtained from a child who is rated in Column A on all 21 items. The highest possible score would be obtained from a child who is rated in Column C on all 21 items.

If the child's score is 24 or less, he is very probably not hyperactive. If the score is 25 to 27, the child *might* be showing a hyperkinetic reac- tion but probably is not. The child can be considered hyperactive and to be showing a hyperkinetic reaction if the score is 28 or higher. He can be considered mildly hyperactive if the score is from 28 to 32, mod- erately hyperactive if the score is from 33 to 37, and severely hyperac- tive if the score is from 38 to 42.

APPROACHES TO TREATMENT

Because hyperactivity can reflect various underlying disorders, a medical diagnosis helps to clarify the nature of your child's difficulties. Appropriate medical treatment for conditions that can cause symptoms which appear to be hyperactivity can then be obtained. For this reason the physician becomes an important professional helper. It is also the physician who can prescribe medication, if that form of treatment is desired.

Your child can't be understood or helped in isolation, because the hyperactivity affects your entire family. Your family may need help in understanding hyperactivity and in dealing with the difficulties that occur within your child and within the other family members. For this reason the mental health professional also becomes a potentially valuable helper. In addition, some of your child's hyperactivity is probably a reflection of the emotional stress that he is experiencing. Direct therapeutic work with your child or indirect reaching of your child through the process of parent counseling or family counseling can often help reduce the hyperactivity.

One of the fastest growing methods of treating hyperactivity is a form of prevention through managing the child's food selection and food intake. The Feingold nutritional program has recently enjoyed much popularity, and it is the major alternative to prescribed medication.

Counseling, nutrition management, and prescribed medication are the three most prominent methods of treatment, and each is considered in this section. In the author's experience, the most effective treatment involves counseling of relevant family members in addition to either the Feingold nutritional program or prescribed medication. To use only one of the three is usually less effective.

Chapter 2

Counseling and Medical Treatment

Most parents of hyperactive children find that medication or nutrition management alone does not solve all of the difficulties of hyperactivity. They discover, too, that a solely behavioral approach, which assumes only psychological causes and discounts the role of medical causes is often inadequate. Most families with hyperactive children can profit from help from both types of resources, because both factors are usually involved. There is usually a biochemical basis for at least some of the hyperactivity, and at least some of it is magnified by psychological factors. In addition, the other family members sometimes react to the hyperactivity in harmful ways that create additional problems.

No single field of knowledge has all of the answers about hyperactivity. Medical and mental health sources of assistance can form a diagnostic and treatment team. Ideally the two sources of help will communicate and cooperate with each other in a united effort.

Both resources should have up-to-date information. Written records and communications often help to avoid misunderstandings that can occur when messages are exchanged only verbally.

Your role as facilitator of these sources of help can be difficult, especially if the professional helpers in your community do not give you credit for knowing much about hyperactivity. You must be assertive without being offensive, insistent without being pushy, and confident without being overbearing. The helpers want to exercise their unique skills for the benefit of your child, and you must give them the freedom to do just that. On the other hand, it is important that you make the final decision in obtaining a satisfactory and truly helpful combination of medical and mental health resources.

Do not stand in awe of people who have many years of college and who have initials after their names. They are human and are capable of making mistakes; they are also capable of being inconsiderate of your feelings. Not every potential helper will be receptive to your diagnosis

43

of hyperactivity in your child, and even fewer will have any idea what to do about it. Use great caution, and be willing to consider other helpers until you find those with whom you feel comfortable.

The professional helpers may assist each other in diagnosis and treatment. The mental health specialist can sometimes be helpful to the physician in the early stages of diagnosis. Sometimes a physician will ask that the family try counseling first before treating the hyperactivity medically. Such an approach provides opportunities for the family members to understand the various patterns of relationships that have developed. The mental health specialist can also help to monitor the behavioral effects of the treatment approach by reporting updated information to the physician. It is not unusual that a mental health professional provides counseling services while a physician provides consultation to the parents with regard to medication or nutrition management.

Be willing to spend several weeks or several months in determining the extent of your child's difficulties and the levels of his abilities. Don't stop the diagnosis process if one of the resource persons claims to have diagnosed all of your child's difficulties. Don't surrender the advantages of the team approach for the apparent simplicity of a one-sided diagnosis and treatment.

Sometimes one of the resources is not much needed and therefore is of only minor assistance. There might be no need for elaborate medical diagnostic procedures or for extensive family counseling. If the child responds well to medication or to nutrition management and if there are few residual family stresses after this favorable response to treatment, the need for helping resources is reduced.

Getting Medical Help for Your Child

Your family's physician or your child's pediatrician may engage the help of supporting persons such as psychiatrists, opthalmologists, or other medical specialists. To find the extent of the hyperactivity, the physician will ask about your child's symptoms. Reports from teachers, sitters, and others who have been able to observe your child will be helpful.

It is important to obtain a thorough medical diagnosis in order to detect underlying conditions which may be responsible for the hyperactivity. Rushing into a premature masking of the symptoms by medication is not good medical practice and makes no sense. Since hyperactivity may have more than one cause in any specific child, thorough diagnostic procedures are doubly important.

To diagnose the hyperactivity the physician should start with a routine physical examination and a medical history interview. The individual methods and aspects of examination and history-taking vary widely among different physicians, and the specific requirements for a thorough diagnosis of your child may be different from the requirements for diagnosis of another child.

For most hyperactive children, the role of the medical helper is to give routine medical service and perhaps to prescribe and monitor treatment of the hyperactivity, either by medication or by nutrition management. Unfortunately, mental health and academic issues are often not addressed until the hyperactivity has had harmful effects. The physician, whose only function is to prescribe medication while the child is not being helped by other needed resources, may be giving treatment that is too narrow to overcome the effects of the hyperactivity.

In order to maintain a good working relationship, give the physician complete and accurate information about the child and about your family. Discuss your concerns about diagnosis and treatment. Do not alter the treatment without consulting the physician.

Getting Mental Health Help for Your Family

The major helper is a professionally qualified mental health specialist, usually a psychologist, social worker, or psychiatrist. Occasionally persons who are counselors or members of the clergy have sufficient training and skill to provide the mental health help for your family. Supporting helpers include other mental health specialists, physicians, educational specialists, speech therapists, and others who advise the major helper. Additional sources of mental health services include foster homes and residential treatment centers.

Sometimes a mental health specialist can provide crucial help to families with a hyperactive child. He can help diagnose and treat the effects of the hyperactivity on the entire family. The mental health specialist will know about hyperactivity as it typically affects families and will assist the other helpers, such as the physician. He can balance the effects of the hyperactivity against various other factors that affect family members.

In some circumstances, standard procedures can be used to measure your child's skills and characteristics. Psychological tests should be given only by persons who have sufficient training and experience in the complicated techniques of administering, scoring, and interpreting them; these skills are usually confined to psychologists. If the major helper is not qualified to provide these services, a psychologist can administer the tests and interpret the results to the major helper or to you. The tests that are most often used in evaluation of hyperactive children measure intelligence, eye-hand coordination, language ability, reading skill, academic knowledge, and personality traits. The specific combination of tests that is needed for your child may differ from that which may be needed for another.

The role of the mental health specialist is not to replace other forms of help and not to explain away the hyperactivity through social causes, but to help the family counter the destructive effects of wrestling with the child's hyperactivity.

As part of the diagnostic phase of help, the mental health specialist will probably take a routine family history, emphasizing your child's social, emotional, and physical development. The purpose of these diagnostic steps is to pave the way for change in the methods by which the family members settle conflicts and express their needs toward each other. If this type of help appears to be needed, a mental health specialist should be sought.

Chapter 3

Treatment by Nutrition Management

The concept of controlling food intake to improve happiness and health is an ancient one, and new plans for food choices and meal schedules are announced often, with much fanfare and in great numbers, but with little scientific backing. Dr. Ben Feingold has developed a program for nutritional control of hyperactivity which has considerable support among the tens of thousands of parents who have adopted it. The medical community has been taking a wait-and-see attitude, but more and more physicians appear to be exploring this method as research, which is still in the early stages, continues to verify its effectiveness. The food and food-chemical industries have generally remained in opposition to it, apparently concerned with their huge investments in methods of food production, storage, shipment, marketing, and promotion.

The Feingold program involves the elimination of all artificial colors and flavors, the preservatives BHA and BHT, and the flavor enhancer MSG. Various other substances are also eliminated, depending on the degree of the child's sensitivity to them. These other substances include salicylates and various food additives. Salicylates are the acidic substances that give many fruits their tangy, bittersweet taste.

According to Dr. Feingold, the elimination of these substances results in significant improvement in a large number of cases. The success rate varies in different research projects. Dr. Feingold cites data indicating that over 50 percent of the hyperactive children placed on the program show significant decrease in hyperactivity. He has found that in many instances in which the program has not been effective, the child has been ingesting an irritating substance. Stricter controls by the parents have often brought about improvement.

After the initial phase in which all of the potentially irritating substances are eliminated and the hyperactivity decreases, the foods containing salicylates can be reintroduced one at a time. They are given in liberal amounts at the rate of one new food item for each four or five days. As time goes on, more and more food items are taken off the forbidden list. Some hyperactive children are found not to be sensitive to any of the foods containing salicylates.

This procedure of replacing suspected food items one at a time allows the offending chemical to be identified quickly. If hyperactivity dramatically reappears when the child is receiving a particular food containing a salicylate, that food item is eliminated *permanently* from the child's diet.

In addition to the elimination and gradual reintroduction of potentially irritating food substances, the Feingold approach also involves a high intake of proteins and a low intake of carbohydrates and sugars. Sometimes this program is used along with standard procedures for the control of allergy and hypoglycemia.

The Prevalence of Carbohydrates and Food Additives

Although the body has no need for refined sugar, carbohydrates are important. They help produce energy, especially for the nervous system, and they help in the metabolism of fats. Natural carbohydrates are generally more useful to the body than refined carbohydrates; natural grains, fruit, and vegetables are considered wholesome sources of needed carbohydrates.

Dr. Feingold's concern about carbohydrates in general and refined sugar in particular is based on some shocking realities. Hyperactive children seem to increase in distractibility, fidgetiness, and other symptoms if their diet is high in carbohydrates. High carbohydrate consumption is also known to contribute to many medical conditions: diabetes, obesity, and stomach problems are the most common ones. Even schizophrenia has been connected by some researchers with high intake of carbohydrates.

Pure granulated sugar is exactly that. It has no vitamins, minerals, or proteins left in it. It is habit-forming, so that the more it is consumed, the more it is craved. The average American consumes 125 pounds of sugar each year, which is equivalent to four-fifths of a cup each day. Sugar accounts for about one-sixth of the average daily diet in terms of total volume. Much of the sugar is contained in other foods, so that even an attempt to limit the use of sugar at the table may not result in much of a decrease in consumption.

Four thousand chemicals have been labeled as drugs by the medical community. An additional twenty-five hundred chemicals are used for flavoring, nutritional supplementation, and coloring in food. Three thousand other chemicals are used as preservatives. Usually, only the additives used in the final stages of food processing are listed on product labels. Synthetic additives occur in about 80 percent of the food items in a typical supermarket. They have no nutritional value and serve only a cosmetic function. Each year the average American eats and drinks over five pounds of additives. According to conservative estimates, some children are eating over one quarter of a pound of coal-tar dyes each year.

The infiltration of additives into common foods is illustrated by such a seemingly innocent product as ice cream. Ice cream can contain diethyl glycol (substitute for eggs), used in antifreeze and paint remover; piperonal (substitute for vanilla), used for killing lice; aldehyde C_{17} (cherry flavor), a flammable liquid used in dyes, plastics, and rubber; and four chemicals (artificial pineapple, nut, banana, and strawberry flavors) which are found in cleaning fluids, rubber cement, and oil paint solvent! Of course the use of a small quantity of a chemical as a flavoring does not have the same effect as the use of a large quantity of the same substance in a nonfood item. Nevertheless, the fact remains that additives seem to be appearing in more and more food items.

An additional difficulty is that some artificial flavors contain over one hundred ingredients, and the formulas produced by competing chemical companies often vary slightly from each other. Thus the monitoring and comparison of artificial flavors and their ingredients are almost impossible tasks.

The Prevalence of Salicylates

A hyperactive child may be found to be sensitive to none, a few, or many of these items which contain salicylates: almonds, apples, apricots, aspirin, bell peppers, all berries, cherries, chili powder, cloves, coffee, cucumbers, currants, grapes, nectarines, oranges, peaches, peppermint and spearmint, pickles, plums, pomegranates, prunes, raisins, tea, and tomatoes.

Advantages of Treatment by Nutrition Management

1. The program does not have some of the disadvantages of treatment by prescribed medication. There is no worry about side effects, no expensive schedule of visits to the physician for renewal of the treatment, no medication to buy, and no worry about unknown long-term effects of the medication.
2. Essential nutrients are not eliminated. The permitted foods form a balanced diet. The eliminated foods are replaced by permitted healthful items.
3. This approach merits consideration by parents of very young hyperactive children for whom medication is likely to have inconsistent, unpredictable, or adverse effects.
4. The program can be maintained unobtrusively in public because the permitted foods are not rare or unusual and there are no bottles or pills to carry.
5. This approach allows the child to develop a sense of responsibility by participation in the control and improvement of behavior through the natural processes of strengthening the body and monitoring food intake. There is no dependence on an external source of needed chemicals.
6. The entire family can join the hyperactive child in the modified food choices. Thus the child will feel less different than would be the case with prescribed medication.
7. There is no clock-watching, and there is no need to coordinate daily schedules and deadlines for administering the treatment.

Concerns About This Method of Treatment

Grocery Shopping

Parents must read the labels on every food product the child will be served, because there can be variations in additives in different brands of a specific food. The recipe for a specific brand may also change, causing the product to be no longer acceptable for the child.

Some products may contain more than one potentially offending chemical. The child may react to a certain brand of catsup, for example, not because of the tomato content (a salicylate) but because of the cloves (another salicylate). Switching to a different brand may allow the child to reintroduce catsup into his regular food choices. Had the parents not carefully noted all of the ingredients, they might have mistakenly considered tomatoes the food item that contributed to the continuing hyperactivity.

The list of ingredients found on the packages or labels of some foods is often not complete, which adds to the difficulty. Manufacturers are under no obligation to make it complete. Among the incompletely labeled items are many standardized products, including bread, cheese, chocolate, cocoa, cornmeal, cream, flour, fruit juices, canned fruits, jams and jellies, macaroni products, mayonnaise, milk, salad dressings, and tomato products.

Dr. Feingold advises parents to keep a record in which the brand names and other important information about all food consumed by the child are entered. Any increase in hyperactivity may then be traced to the intake of an irritating chemical to which the child is sensitive. With a little practice, a shopping list of safe food can be developed. There is no need to shop at natural food stores; permitted items are available at regular food markets. Because only a small minority of hyperactive children seem to be bothered by the salicylates, the fruits and vegetables containing salicylates can usually be reintroduced into the child's diet in a few months.

In addition to careful shopping for food, similar precautions must be taken when buying medicines. When it comes in a colored capsule, only the white powder inside may be nonirritating to the child's system. Most children's medicine contains artificial flavoring or coloring. The medical services departments of drug companies will provide information on the ingredients in their products to concerned parents. Pharmacists and physicians are additional sources of guidance in the choice of medicines for the salicylate-sensitive child's use. A list of some additive-free medicines currently available is given in the Appendices.

Planning and Preparing Meals

Because of the elimination of preprocessed (often *over*-processed) foods, many of the so-called convenience products must not be used.

For some parents, this change is hard to make. There is no avoiding the fact that it takes time and effort to prepare nutritious, home-cooked meals. The single parent who must work outside the home each day in addition to assuming the homemaking and cooking responsibilities for the family may find the switch away from preprocessed food a difficult challenge. Items like donuts, candy, and ice cream are usually prohibited unless made from special recipes at home. Some parents, though, are surprised to find that they can prepare items at home which they thought were available only from stores.

For many families, a nutrition management program does not change their eating habits, just their choice of brands. Once the shopping routine becomes established, meal preparation also takes less time. Home-prepared food is, of course, more nutritious and better tasting than preprocessed food.

Making Eating Out Preparations

When the family is traveling, special care will probably have to be taken in selecting restaurants. In some cases, food should be prepared at home prior to the trip. Most restaurants serve highly processed food without regard to its additive content. Vegetarian restaurants and cafeterias can sometimes be handy sources of permitted food. In other restaurants, a polite request to know the brands or check the labels of the items that are being offered will usually be honored if it is explained that the child is sensitive to certain food chemicals.

Maintaining the Program

One food violation can trigger a hyperactive reaction in some children within minutes. Two or three violations per week can keep the child in a constant hyperactive state. The motto for food that is unknown to the parent or that is incompletely labeled is: When in doubt, avoid it.

Monitoring and supervision are vital. They become increasingly difficult as the child grows older, especially if the child starts to become uncooperative, or as he eats more often at friends' homes or at restaurants.

The fact that minor alterations of food intake can switch the hyperactivity on and off is reassuring; it proves the accuracy of this approach. The challenge for the family is to provide the structure and supervision that will be helpful but inoffensive for the child. Parents should eliminate needless temptations like additive-laden snack items and similar products commonly known as junk food. Helping the child become aware of the positive effects of the program can prevent violations. Parents can make the child aware of the before and after contrasts in behavior and achievements. Parents must accommodate gracefully to occasional infractions by the child, emphasizing the positive changes in him when the program is observed. The program should be started at a time when parents have complete control, during a long weekend or a school vacation period, for example. The child will gradually become proud of the new method of self-control and violations will begin to decrease.

The child can be invited to join in label reading. Any anger that he may feel in response to the rigid control of his food intake will then be directed toward the forbidden product rather than toward the parents who prohibit it.

Some attention needs to be given to persons outside the family who may mistakenly offer forbidden items to the child. Parents should explain the program to the parents of the child's friends and playmates, to sitters, to members of the family, and to any others who may need to know about it. Sending an additive-free snack from home with the child when he is visiting a friend is a simple method that works well for many parents.

Supervision at School

Parties at school pose a special challenge for hyperactive children who are participating in treatment by nutrition management. Ask the teacher to send a note or to call home to inform you of upcoming parties. You can then send acceptable substitutes for the treats that other children receive. The teacher may also be willing to encourage certain fruits, nuts, or additive-free treats for the entire class as a more healthful alternative to ordinary sweets.

The school lunch period is the most likely time of day for the child to violate his nutrition program. There may be pressure from classmates to share their additive-laden food and desserts, which are offered as gestures of friendship. Your child may be tempted to sell his lunch ticket or to trade lunches with classmates. He may have access to vending machines with disallowed food in them. If your child is intent on violating the treatment program, the teacher has only to turn his or her back for a few seconds in order for him to succeed. Cafeteria supervision is difficult because teachers usually rotate lunch supervision duty and because they may be supervising hundreds of children at the same time. Unless the school provides lunches that meet the requirements of the nutrition management program, you will have to send the lunch from home with the child, or arrange for him to return home or to a trusted neighbor for lunch.

Detecting Environmental Irritants

Some very sensitive children will not show a substantial reduction in hyperactivity, even with careful application of the Feingold nutritional program. In many cases that at first appear unsuccessful with this method of treatment, the child is absorbing offending substances by some means other than food intake. Irritating molecules might be inhaled, or they might be absorbed through the skin. A thorough check for potentially offending substances of this type can sometimes uncover sources of stimulation for the child's hyperactivity that would otherwise have been overlooked. While not actually part of the Feingold nutritional program, the survey for environmental irritants has been helpful to many parents who were not experiencing the degree of success they had expected from the program.

Table 2 lists the types of irritants that appear to stimulate reactions in hyperactive children.

TABLE 2   Examples of Environmental Irritants that Can Trigger an Increase in the Hyperactivity of an Exposed Child

Clothing
any polyester fabric or item
polyester bedding
permanent press clothes not yet washed
TRIS flame retardant in clothes

House fixtures
blown-in insulation with urea-formaldehyde

smell from new carpeting
fluorescent lighting
oil, natural gas, and coal heating systems
propane appliances
vinyl wallpaper
interior of new mobile homes
glue used in flooring, wallpaper, and paneling

TABLE 2 (Continued)

Playthings
ball-point ink on skin
invisible ink on skin
felt-tip marker on skin
colored chalk
chalk dust in the air
finger paint
scratch and sniff books
putty-like, slimy, and clay-like
   modeling compounds
caps and fireworks
white powder inside balloons
Easter-egg dye

Toiletries
alcohol on skin
hand lotion
colored and perfumed soap
facial powder
eye shadow
fingernail polish
lipsticks to prevent chapping
perfume
after-shave lotion
hair spray
toothpaste
bubble bath
dental cleaning agents
fluoride treatment
adhesive bandages
colored and flavored medicine

Cleaning and polishing agents
disinfectant containing methyl salicylate
pine fragrance soap
furniture and floor wax
oven cleaner
pine fragrance liquid cleaner

rug shampoo
colored dishwasher detergent
fabric softener sheets for dryer

Paper products
colored or scented paper towels
colored or scented facial tissue
colored or scented bathroom
   tissue
colored cupcake liners
paper wiping rags

Workshop chemicals
fumes of paint, varnish, etc.
glue (including postage stamps
   and envelope seals)
gasoline fumes
gasoline or oil leak
chlorine in swimming pool
airborne particles of paint or varnish from sanding finished
   wood
freshly poured blacktop

Aromatics
mothballs
incense
scented candle
air freshener
dog and cat repellent
aerosol spray cans
smoke from a fire
smoke from a menthol cigarette

Plastics
old teflon pans, flaking
polyurethane food-storage bowls
plastic food wrap
waterbeds

In summary, the concerns and objections that have been raised about using this method of treatment include these:

1. it is not yet entirely accepted by the professional medical community;
2. not all children have responded favorably to this method;
3. it involves more effort at planning and preparing meals than some families are accustomed to;
4. it eliminates many convenience and snack food items;
5. it is difficult to ensure that the child will follow the program without being directly supervised by adults, at least at first;
6. restaurants usually are not used to accommodating to such a program;
7. food shopping becomes more painstaking at first than some families are accustomed to;
8. food shopping must involve constant label reading of food products.

Some parents lack the maturity to sacrifice their personal whims for the sake of the child's development; these parents will no doubt find ways to circumvent the program. Others seem unable to make the necessary arrangements in their lives despite a sincere interest in this method. Still others find that, despite earnest application, this approach is ineffective for their child. For these groups of parents, treatment by prescribed medication usually becomes the preferred method.

Getting Support from Others

This nutritional method is a recent development, and many physicians and mental health professionals still doubt its effectiveness, in part because only limited research has been reported in the professional journals.

School personnel may be hesitant about accommodating to the child's program for a variety of reasons. Parents may feel awkward about explaining the program to friends or relatives, for fear of being misunderstood or ridiculed.

Regular contact with other parents who are using this program provides a sense of support. Feingold Associations have formed in many communities. They offer group support and sponsor educational programs about hyperactivity. They develop shopping guides and food lists geared to their specific localities, based on the combined shopping experiences of member families. They also distribute recipes for preparing approved food items.

Through the efforts of such organizations, an antihistamine decongestant that is free of artificial ingredients has been developed. Colorless and naturally flavored candy has also been developed through Feingold Association activity. Other common projects include newsletters, negotiating with school systems about changing school lunch policies, and finding meat processors and dairies that will produce their items without the usual additives.

A list of active Feingold Associations appears in the Appendices of this book, together with suggestions for further reading on additive-free cooking and the Feingold nutritional program.

Chapter 4

Treatment by Prescribed Medication

The most frequently used types of medication are stimulants and antidepressants. Children whose hyperactivity stems from profound mental illness, anxiety, or severe damage to the brain through infection or injury may need other forms of medication.

Amphetamines (Dexedrine, for example) and methylphenidate (Ritalin) are the most frequently used stimulants. Caffeine is also known to assist in controlling hyperactivity.

Antidepressants such as imipramine (Tofranil, for example) tend to be longer lasting in their effect than stimulants. They are sometimes prescribed so that only one dose is required each day, in contrast to the two or three doses per day required of stimulants. Antidepressants are often given when bed wetting is one of the child's difficulties.

Tranquilizers are another kind of medication that is sometimes prescribed. If the hyperactivity is caused by underlying emotional disturbance, tranquilizers produce improvement. A tranquilizer given to a child whose hyperactivity is not psychologically caused, however, merely worsens the symptoms. The hyperactive child who gets worse when given a tranquilizer probably is not hyperactive as a result of underlying anxiety or emotional disturbance.

It may appear strange that medication which stimulates would be used to create calmness in an already overly aroused child. These medications, however, tend to stimulate the child's brain to block out irrelevant thought and to focus attention. In a sense, these medications stimulate the child's mental "brake pedal" rather than the child's mental "gas pedal." The exact site of chemical activity is not yet agreed upon by researchers, and various parts of the brain have been suggested as possible locations affected by these medications.

Factors Affecting Treatment by Medication

The age of the child, the timing of administration of the medication, and the dosage are the three chief factors which determine how effective the medication will be.

Age of the Child

Experience has shown that the most predictable results from these medications occur with hyperactive children who are between the ages of six and twelve. In children younger than six or older than twelve there is a greater tendency for side effects to be prominent and for the desired results to be less potent.

Among children whose hyperactivity continues to be obvious during adolescence, there may be several reasons for the decreased effectiveness of medication. The hyperactive adolescent is better able to undermine the treatment by outright refusal to cooperate. He is also more likely to be purposeful in outward behavior, more or less in spite of medication. The desire for adolescent rebellion may propel the hyperactive teenager into continued misbehavior despite any increase in ability to focus attention or use sound judgment.

Timing

During warm weather, children are more active and have less need for concentrated attention. Physicians sometimes will ask that medication be discontinued at those times. Removal of the medication during the summer also minimizes the slight stunting of growth that may sometimes occur as a side effect.

The child is medicated usually in the morning and at noon, with additional doses occasionally prescribed for the afternoon or the late evening. Late evening doses are sometimes prescribed in an attempt to control bed wetting. To counteract early morning irritability, the morning dose is sometimes given while the child is still in bed, about thirty minutes before the regular time to get up. Parents and teachers sometimes notice that a medicated hyperactive child will show a clear deterioration in behavior late in the afternoon. In these cases, the medication is losing its effect; a slightly higher dose for morning or noon is usually helpful, but only with the physician's approval.

Dosage

Factors such as the child's general activity level, history of disease, current medical status, age, height, weight, and severity of hyperactivity are considered in deciding what dosage to prescribe. Most knowledgeable physicians start the medication at a low dosage level, gradually increasing it until the maximum desired effect is reached. The dosage indicators in Table 3 are often used.

TABLE 3   Dosage Indicators

Child's Behavior	Dosage Adjustment
Hyperactivity	Increase dosage
Absence of most hyperactive tendencies	Increase dosage slightly, or maintain current level
Drowsy, appears drugged, sleepy at school, loss of appetite	Reduce dosage slightly
Works furiously for hours, compulsive, intense	Reduce dosage greatly, consider tranquilizer, or discontinue all medication
Seeing or hearing things which are not present, constant talking, euphoric, on a high	Reduce dosage greatly, consider tranquilizer, or discontinue all medication

During the first few days of medication, no change may occur in the child's behavior. The physician will then slowly increase the dosage until some change occurs. The dosage can then be increased gradually until the first indications of drowsiness appear; then the dosage can be adjusted slightly downward. In this way, the physician can be guided to a dosage that provides the maximum desired effect with minimum side effect.

Advantages of Treatment by Medication

1. Giving medication involves no change in family habits of shopping, meal planning, food preparation, or food choices.
2. Treatment can take place anywhere because of the portability of pills. It can continue when the family is travelling, when the child is

away from home, and in other circumstances where nutrition management would be awkward or difficult.

3. It is easier to enforce. The parent can supervise the taking of the medication, so that even if not convinced of the benefits of treatment, the child can nevertheless be prevented from hindering it.

Concerns About This Method of Treatment

Medication vs. Drug Abuse

Some parents fear that their child may become addicted to the medication. They may also be concerned that the child would be more likely to abuse drugs in the future or that the child would lose mental alertness.

There are important differences between illegal use of black-market drugs and appropriately monitored use of medication prescribed by a physician. Drug abuse and consequent addiction are usually created by constant overuse of a medication without medical supervision. These medications do not create addiction when prescribed in appropriate doses for hyperactive children. Hyperactive children do not crave medication; in fact, they often oppose taking it. They usually do not ask to receive it again after it has been discontinued. They experience no euphoria or high from it. When appropriately prescribed, administered, and monitored, these medications help to prevent the problems that would otherwise propel these children into the drug-abusing subculture. Only those children who are receiving incorrectly prescribed dosage levels appear significantly drugged.

Side Effects

The medication sometimes produces these side effects: nervousness, difficulty sleeping, irritability, headache, restlessness, nail biting, drowsiness, cold hands and feet, appetite loss, skin rash, or slight stunting of growth.

Most of these potential side effects are controlled by adjustments in dosage or by a switch to a different type of medication. Appetite loss can be countered by having the child eat meals before rather than after taking the medication. Skin rash can be stopped by discontinuing the medication for a few days, until the rash disappears, then beginning it again.

Additional side effects are possible for any individual child, and there has been little systematic study of long-term side effects.

Maintaining This Method

Some of these medications are popular among drug-abusing adolescents and adults, who obtain them illegally and consume them in large amounts; consequently, some parents are concerned that their child may try to sell the medication to classmates or playmates, either out of personal choice or under pressure from the other children. To avoid this circumstance, the medicine should be in a protected and, if necessary, locked place and should be under the parents' direct control. Medication at school should also be under adult supervision.

The child should be helped to find ways to take the medication discreetly and privately when in a public place, at a social occasion, or at school. Many children are embarrassed about having to take medicine and resent their dependency on it.

Parents and teachers should monitor the child's behavior and watch for side effects. Periodic reports to the physician can help to determine adjustments of the dosage.

The administration of the medication should be kept on a prescribed schedule. Misplacing the bottle or losing track of time can cause disruption in the treatment for the day. The prescription and the clock necessarily become important factors in the daily lives of the child and the parent.

In summary, the concerns and objections that have been raised about using this method of treatment include these:

1. long-term study of side effects has not been done, so the safety of this method is less certain than the safety of nutrition management;
2. dosage level is determined by loose criteria and can be influenced by personal bias of the physician;
3. some children are overmedicated and appear drugged, and parents have no guarantee that this will not happen to their child;
4. there is a danger that the medication will attract drug abusers to the child;
5. this method risks psychological dependence by the child on external chemicals;
6. the medication must be supervised and kept in controlled or locked locations;

7. the child has to find unobtrusive opportunities for taking the medication when away from home, to avoid embarrassment;

8. this method is not considered effective for children of preschool age or younger.

Medication vs. Nutrition Management: Pros and Cons

The two methods can be compared in several ways, so that the most appropriate method for any particular family can be selected.

• SIMPLICITY. Prescribed medication is less time-consuming than nutrition management. Nutrition management, however, eliminates clock-watching. Grocery shopping becomes simplified, after a while, under nutrition management, because parents learn exactly which grocery products to buy and are therefore less subject to impulse buying at the market.

• EFFECTIVENESS. Research data are not conclusive about either method, but the overall trend seems to be that at least half of the children treated with either method respond with significant improvement while about one in four respond somewhat favorably. With both methods, about one in four children seem not to respond favorably to the treatment. Sometimes a child who will not respond favorably to one method will do so to the other method.

• SECURITY. Nutrition management is easier than treatment by medication for the child to disrupt. Parental supervision of medication guarantees that the child is following the treatment program. A violation of food guidelines, however, is possible whenever the child is near forbidden food and out of the parents' view.

• SAFETY. The two methods are probably both safe, though there is more suspicion about the safety of medication because its long-term effects have not been studied thoroughly. Use of medication does not lead to drug abuse, and no side effects have been proved damaging to the health of children who take the medication. The nutrition management method is free of any questionable substances and involves a wholesome and balanced selection of food.

• ECONOMY. Nutrition management is the more economical method. There is no medicine to purchase, and there is usually no need for periodic visits to the physician. The required food items are not exotic or expensive. Further economy is introduced because preprocessed and junk food—usually expensive types of groceries—are eliminated.

• PSYCHOLOGICAL EFFECT. Medication is more likely to train the child to look to outside sources as the causes and cures for life's problems. Nutrition management involves the natural act of eating wholesome food and teaches the child to take care of himself.

• EMBARRASSMENT. Either method is potentially embarrassing to the child if not handled with care. Medicine should be given unobtrusively and in private, and nutrition management should be done with attention to the child's need for a well-rounded food assortment, including desserts.

• ISOLATION. In a family that can follow the nutrition guidelines, the child is less likely to feel singled out as different when nutrition management is used.

• POPULAR ACCEPTABILITY. Food sensitivity has more popular acceptance by adults than the need for medication. The general public distrusts the widespread use of behavior-controlling medication. The idea of keeping a child's sugar intake low and feeding the child additive-free food is much less offensive. To the professional medical community, however, treatment by nutrition management is suspect while medication is more accepted.

Which Method for Your Child?

Neither method cures hyperactivity. When either method is discontinued, the result is an immediate reappearance of the hyperactivity. Both methods involve adherence to certain substances; any deviation causes a return of the disorder. Both methods have strong proponents and strong opponents. Research findings have not conclusively shown that medication side effects are harmless, nor have they shown the Feingold nutritional program to be consistently effective.

In the long run, medication appears to be more expensive and more risky. We must be aware of the potency of these medications and acknowledge that there is some risk in using anything about which there is less than full knowledge. Nutrition management involves eliminating additive-laden food and establishing a staple diet of wholesome food. There is no introduction of questionable substances into the child's body, and there is no worry about long-term side effects.

Each family must make its own decision about the method of treatment, based on careful weighing of advantages and disadvantages of each method. Parents who conclude that adjustments in meal preparation and shopping are too cumbersome, or who prefer a method that makes it harder for the child to cheat, will probably choose medication as the method of treatment.

SECTION THREE

FEELINGS AND RELATIONSHIPS IN YOUR FAMILY

The hardest struggles take place within your heart. The tortuous emotional roller coaster that you as the parent have experienced is discussed in this section, along with your child's inner struggles.

The stress of a child's hyperactivity exerts a predictable force on the parents' marital relationship. The consistent patterns of marital discord that seem to occur most often among parents of hyperactive children are explained, and numerous suggestions are given for preventing those patterns and for improving the situation if they have already started to occur.

Your child's relations with brothers and sisters, classmates, and playmates are also considered in this section. Specific guidelines are given for helping your child improve those relations.

The most common barriers to positive self-esteem among hyperactive children are discussed, and methods of nurturing your child's sense of worth and competence are outlined.

The final chapter in this section suggests remedies for healing your family's emotional wounds, in the form of specific activities that generate love within the family. Love is the universal healer, and it can be regained by use of the methods given here. These activities will be helpful for any family, regardless of the amount of stress or the presence of handicapping conditions among family members. To the extent that your child's hyperactivity is being successfully managed (for example, with the aid of nutrition management or medication), your child will be able to participate with full and sustained effort and enjoyment. The less hyperactive your child is during these activities, the more effective they will be in returning harmony and a sense of family unity to your home.

Chapter 5

Your Child's Self-Esteem

Your Child's Emotional Stresses

It is impossible to understand your child's hyperactivity without first understanding your child's feelings *about* the hyperactivity. Some hyperactive children are optimistic, carefree, and enthusiastic. Your child may have these and other positive feelings and emotions which do not cause stress in your family. These feelings of well-being will not be discussed here. Instead, this chapter outlines the seven most common unpleasant concerns that hyperactive children have:

1. an awareness of being driven
2. a confusion and denial about the hyperactivity
3. an awareness of feeling attacked
4. an awareness of feeling rejected
5. an awareness of being a brat
6. an awareness of being angry toward others
7. an awareness of being angry about himself

Being Driven

Hyperactive children are impulsive and quick to react. They may act as if they are magnetically drawn to situations, events, and people around them—to explore, to touch, to oppose, to question, and to badger. This involvement can appear to be senseless, excessive, automatic, and driven.

Hyperactive children often have a fear of being out of control. They feel helpless to prevent their impulsive acts, even though they know better than to commit them. Sometimes they think of themselves as being two people—a wild or monster self and a calm self.

What to Do: Try to get your child to recognize the condition without either exaggerating or minimizing it. Help your child acknowledge that certain of his actions result from impulsiveness. Without such an awareness, your child may be left with a bizarre explanation for his behavior, such as thinking that he is crazy.

Your child's power to make choices is a key to his ability to get along with others. Treatment by medication or nutrition management will not force him to behave appropriately. It may, however, help to allow him to do so, by making him less driven and more able to make a rational choice of actions.

Too often, however, a hyperactive child is placed in a treatment program without any follow-through responsibility taken by parents, teachers, or the child himself. In some families, the medication or nutrition program ends up being blamed for not being effective enough in preventing recurring misbehavior.

Your child must make consistent effort toward improving his behavior regardless of the effectiveness of the treatment programs. He must be taught that he cannot be excused from helping to set things right after he has misbehaved and that he is responsible for the effects of all his actions, whether driven or not.

Being Unaware

Your child may lack insight into the hyperactivity and may deny that he is hyperactive. Among the abilities that hyperactivity can impair is the ability to make social judgments, including judgments about self. Your child may be psychologically blind to his own hyperactivity.

Hyperactive children are almost always confused and surprised by the negative reactions of others because they do not recognize anything irritating in their own actions.

What to Do: Your child's awareness of his hyperactivity is the key to his ability to understand himself.

Ideally your child should be able to list the things that are difficult for him to do. He should be able to tell you what they are candidly, without emotional upset. The child who can frankly acknowledge that he has difficulty sitting still in school, for example, will be better able to deal with his hyperactivity than the child who is unaware of his traits.

Your child's traits must be acknowledged by *you* without emotional upset. Ideally they should be regarded as differences in your child that are neither good nor bad. They need neither be denied nor defended.

It is more important that your child know what his limitations are than that he know about the label "hyperactive," though there is nothing wrong with using the word hyperactive to describe aspects of your child's behavior. The danger in labeling your child's actions comes from *abuse* of the label; others may use it for name-calling or for embarrassing your child.

A simple method can be used to help make your child aware of his hyperactivity. Immediately after he has acted in a hyperactive fashion, tell your child that you want to help him understand what he is doing. Use a short sentence and speak in a kind but firm tone of voice. Typical statements are these: "This is one of those times"; and "When you do that, I suspect that you are not aware of it."

The method of contrasting also helps. Point out the contrast whenever he is calm in a situation in which he is usually fidgety. Comment on the contrast between your child's current behavior and his ordinarily hyperactive behavior. A typical statement is this: "Usually at these times you are drumming your fingers; it seems easier for you to control yourself today."

Another method is the before/after comparison. After your child is receiving treatment by nutrition management or medication, for example, describe the changes in his behavior.

Being Attacked

It is common for hyperactive children to feel abused by others. The less the child is aware of the nature of his hyperactivity, the more unfair and malicious the criticism from others will seem to be. The child may feel as if he is always in trouble and always being blamed for something. The blaming may come from siblings, friends, teachers, parents, other family members, or even strangers.

The traits for which a hyperactive child can feel blamed are endless. Typical sore points include being criticized for such behavior as:
—being too noisy and making clicks, whistles, and sounds
—being too curious, too inquisitive, asking too many questions
—being too impatient, not waiting for things
—being grabby, wanting to touch, poke, and feel things
—moving around the classrooms at school
—fidgeting, drumming fingers, biting nails, chewing pencils
—being too talkative.

The child may not understand that these criticisms reflect his own hyperactive behavior. He may then simply be bent on revenge. If he is accused of stealing, for example, he may be more concerned about getting back at the tattler than about the moral issues of his stealing. *What to Do:* Try to use the criticisms of others to make your child more aware of his hyperactivity. Only when he understands that these criticisms are based on his own actions can he begin to deal with them constructively. Then he will be less likely to think of others as being unfair or out to get him.

The principle of undoing will help your child develop conscience. One of the most important but difficult lessons for your child to learn is this: He must undo and reverse the negative effects of his actions toward others as soon as possible after the incident has occurred.

Undoing means paying for damage to others' property, with money or with service. It means giving an apology. It means doing surprise favors for others to show the child's desire to improve the situation.

The meaning and purpose of an apology is often a hard concept to teach a hyperactive child. An apology is a lot more than a mechanical "I'm sorry" while being prodded by a parent. It should be done from a position of personal strength, rather than being a self-critical and pathetic appeal for forgiveness. The child should say that he wants to improve his relations with the offended person and that he is willing to do whatever is needed to achieve that. A typical apology is this: "I don't want to have you *not* like me. What can I do to show you that I still want to be your friend?"

Lead your child away from seeking revenge, toward an attitude of forgiveness. Revengeful parents produce revengeful children, and forgiving parents produce forgiving children. By being firm but benevolent when others are unfair, you can do a lot to help your child develop a wholesome attitude toward others.

Being Rejected

Hyperactive children often don't clearly sense the passage of time. As a result, everything starts over with each passing moment. For example, you might not get credit for having just spent a long time with your child. When you announce that you must turn to something else, he may instantly feel neglected and abandoned. The sense of rejection may be the same as it would have been had you not spent any time with him at all.

Your child may conclude that others are purposely not paying attention to him. Even though your child may be bossy and critical and therefore drive others away, he may not see the connection between his actions and the reactions of others.

Your child may eventually conclude that he is unwanted, and possibly hated. He may complain of having no friends and of being unloved within the family.

It is common for hyperactive children to reject others in return. Sometimes they want to leave the neighborhood or run away from home in an attempt to avoid being rejected. They may begin to withdraw from other people and prefer to be alone much of the time.

What to Do: Help your child understand that rejection by others is a result of his own actions. Help him understand that he helps to trigger others' reactions by being abrasive or unpleasant. Without criticizing or preaching, quietly tell him that he has acted in a way that caused others to want to leave him. He needs to become aware of the connection between his moments of hyperactive behavior and others' desire to shun him.

Your child will never learn social skills by avoiding social contact. Don't support your child's attempts to reject others. Instead, encourage him to undo and redeem the situation, so that others do not have hurt feelings and will no longer want to avoid him.

Often it helps to teach your child exactly what to do in a situation in which he runs a risk of being rejected. Give him small, easy steps to take.

Become involved in your child's social life. If you become a group leader in your child's church or scouting organization, he may then participate in such groups, which he might otherwise not be able to join. You can also help your child make improvements in his social behavior within those groups.

Being a Brat

Faced with a constant stream of negative reactions from others, your child may take the path of least resistance. He may decide that those who criticize and reject him are correct and adopt a troublemaker role in the family as well as in the classroom or in the play group. Prevented from being the best, your child may elect to become the best worst in the group.

A brat role is hard to stop once it has started. Numbed by the constant negative responses from others, your child may adopt an "I don't care what you think" attitude. As time goes on, your child may convince himself that he truly does *not* care what others think about how he acts. When he stops caring about others' feelings, he loses an important motivation for remaining socialized.

When competition is carried to an extreme, children tend to become opposites or to be in vivid contrast to each other. Motivated by an intense underlying rivalry toward the hyperactive child, and seeing an opportunity to exploit the inappropriateness of the hyperactive child's behavior, other children can go to great lengths to appear very obedient, cooperative, and innocent. At the same time, they try to make sure that parents and other adults see the marked contrast between their seemingly angelic traits and the brat type of behavior shown by the hyperactive child.

The angel is very much concerned with maintaining his other image and an equally one-sided image of devilishness for the hyperactive child. Whenever your hyperactive child is in a weak or vulnerable position, the angel may be quick to point out that he or she does not do the same kinds of things. The more determined angel may goad, urge, dare, or trick the hyperactive child into misbehaving, then quickly tattle. The angel's ultimate goal is to gain special status with parents and to prove himself or herself in their eyes to be better than the brat. The angel's manipulations are attention-getting misbehavior which is every bit as destructive and inappropriate as the misbehavior of the supposedly devilish hyperactive child.

Your child's friends may try to talk him into doing things that he knows are wrong. When they want to build something, they may say, "Let's use your dad's hammer," and your child may agree to the idea. Your child will end up facing an angered parent, and the other children will escape without suffering any consequences for their actions.

Sometimes the situation is made worse by the hyperactive child, who quickly learns to point out instances in which the sibling is not being angelic. The sibling then tries harder to be a contrast to the hyperactive child. In this way, each of the children becomes more polarized in his or her behavior pattern.

The angel-brat syndrome can eventually develop so that your child becomes the black sheep of the family, classroom, or neighborhood. The hyperactive child can become a scapegoat, the dumping ground for all of the group's or family's stresses, and the whipping boy for frustrated adults.

The wake effect can force your child to stay in a brat role. Think of the child as a speedboat, the hyperactivity as the motor, and the water as the child's relations with others. The motor propels the boat rapidly through the water, splitting and dividing the water. When the motor stops, the boat no longer moves across the water, so will stop splitting the water. However, the wake will catch up with the boat and rock it. In the same way, a hyperactive child builds up a reputation among others that will keep him in a disruptive role long after he stops being hyperactive. The reputation will continue to plague the child, and others will continue to treat him as if he is still a brat, long after he has stopped being one.

When a hyperactive child receives effective treatment by medication or nutrition management, he is often not accepted in his new form. Neighbors and other children are often the last to acknowledge the improvements in the child's behavior. Faced with their expectation that he will still act like a brat, the child may continue in that role despite treatment of the underlying hyperactivity.

Sometimes an aggressive hyperactive child will be successfully treated with medication or nutrition management and will become friendly, cooperative, and kindhearted. The wake, however, will have created enemies among other children who may be eager to get revenge. Thus it is not uncommon for formerly aggressive hyperactive children to be bullied and assaulted during the first few months of successful treatment of their hyperactivity, despite the improvement in their behavior.

Sometimes your child may be afraid to stop being a brat because he may feel pressured if he behaves appropriately for an extended period of time. He may fear that others will *expect* him to continue good behavior. At the same time, he may be afraid of becoming out of control. He may purposely misbehave to make sure that others do not begin to expect that he will maintain good behavior for an extended length of time. A hyperactive child can be as terror-stricken at having to meet others' expectation of showing good behavior, as a normally well-behaved child would if he were expected to misbehave.

What to Do: Try to keep the total situation in mind whenever your child seems to be in trouble with others. Be aware of the motives of the other children. Notice their special interest in tattling on your child or comparing themselves favorably with him. Say something like this: "I wonder if Billy is telling on others so that I will tell him how good he is." Let the children respond to your thought, and encourage them to talk frankly about what is going on.

Notice others' reactions to your child on the basis of his reputation. Urge them instead to react to him on the basis of his current behavior. Watch your own tendency to jump to conclusions about who did it. If your child must go on trial, let the trial be conducted on evidence, not on reputation!

Undoing the wake effect cannot take place until the hyperactivity is successfully managed. From the moment the hyperactivity comes under control, the burden is on your child to demonstrate to others that he is now different. He must prove that he will stop hurting the feelings of others. Help your child understand that others have learned to expect him to act in certain ways, to which they have responded with attacks and rejection. He must now prove to the other children and adults that such hyperactive behavior will no longer occur.

The adults and children in your child's life will probably not believe him when he says he has improved. They will probably continue to react to him as if he were still hyperactive. It may take a year or longer for your child to undo his reputation and convince others to have a better feeling about him. Your child must *show* others that the hyperactive behavior has stopped. At the same time, he must *tell* them of these changes and of his desire to change his relationships.

Your child can make a list of persons who should know of the change and then explain the new situation to each of them. He should also clearly show his desire to demonstrate the improved behavior.

This type of direct undoing of the wake is most effective. If your child is unable to use this method, you can help by talking individually with adults who regularly see your child. Explain the wake effect to them, and tell them of the improvement that is occurring because of treatment of the hyperactivity. Ask them to help undo the wake among your child's classmates and playmates.

Sometimes a direct appeal to the other children can be made. Tell them that your child will be behaving better toward them and that you would like them to treat him with similar respect and kindness. Point out that adults have started to speak in softer tones to him because he misbehaves less often, and state that you want the children to help him see positive results from his improvement.

Being Angry with Others

Hyperactive children often feel abused by others and settle, at least partially, into a troublemaker role. They are angry children, angry with other people as well as with themselves.

The emotions of hyperactive children tend to be extreme. They are usually *very* affectionate or *very* hostile. Changes between these extremes can be rapid, so that these children appear to be moody. One of the causes of these extreme and rapidly changing moods is that hyperactive children find it hard to express their needs and emotions in words. Instead, they let their emotions build up, then discharge them through extreme and impulsive action. Typically, they have a short fuse and a bad temper. They may explode in fits of rage that endanger others' safety. They may break windows, punch holes through walls, kick doors, knock over furniture, and attack others with knives. The anger of hyperactive children, like their other emotions, tends to fluctuate greatly and to be extreme. When the anger is expressed in words, it is often by needling, teasing, and picking on other children.

Hyperactive children sometimes show their anger in a competitive attitude. Like most competitive persons, hyperactive children who are competitive are poor winners and poor losers. If they win, they make fun of the loser and flaunt their victory in an overbearing way; if they are about to lose, they may demand a rule change or quit the activity. If they do lose, they may accuse the opponent of cheating and may even attack him.

What to Do: Teach your child to negotiate with others rather than having fits of rage. Your child can learn to come to a helping adult, state that he is angry, and tell the adult what he is angry about. The adult can then suggest some possible solutions. Another method is for your child to write down what he is angry about and discuss it at the end of the day. Both of these methods teach your child to:

1. withdraw from the situation rather than attack people;
2. translate anger into words rather than tantrums;
3. report the feelings to a concerned adult.

Both methods depend on the availability of a calm, helpful adult.

Teaching your child to leave the scene when he feels angry is not the best solution because it does not permit practice at using social skills to change the situation. It is, however, a starting point for change in behavior. Leaving the scene can allow your child to cool off and regain control over his emotions.

Having an old mattress for jumping on and a punching bag for hitting will give your child a chance to vent anger, and will prevent useless and destructive attacks on people and objects. However, because this method does not teach improved social skills, it is not a good long-range solution.

The best long-range answer to the problem of your child's anger is to teach him how to deal with other people in conflict situations. A simple procedure will give him the basic tools. Your child should use this procedure whenever he starts to become uncomfortable with what others are doing, before he builds up anger. Teach your child to say "That bothers me; please stop it" or "I don't want you to do that to me." This procedure gives your child experience at saying immediately and directly how he feels, and to ask clearly for what he wants.

Being Angry with Self

Hyperactivity is frustrating for your child. He is aware that others consider him disruptive. Any amount of hyperactivity provides fuel for self-criticism. Your child may realize that he can't pay attention to one thing for very long and does not follow through on projects. He may regret that he is unable to sit quietly and to read a whole chapter in a book without stopping. He may be angry at himself for not being able to do neatly written work at school. He may be disgusted at his clumsiness, often destroying or breaking whatever he touches.

Your child may start to feel unhappy about his difficulty in expressing feelings, thoughts, and desires. He may realize that others think of him as domineering.

He may feel ignorant and incompetent, with self-applied labels like dumb and stupid, considering himself a misfit who is a disgrace and who does not belong in the family.

Ultimately he may not be able to accept positive feelings and messages about himself, tending to discount or explain away any success or any compliment given to him by others. Wallowing in self-hatred, your child may become bitterly unhappy and pessimistic about himself and about life.

What to Do: Help your child increase his feelings of self-esteem by showing your appreciation for his strengths and positive traits. Make encouraging remarks about his capabilities and his importance to you. Have your child practice the skills that he is concerned about. In this way, he can gain confidence as his skills improve. Practice should be done in a light-hearted supportive atmosphere rather than one of coercion or pressure. When possible, work practice into play activities. The child who has difficulty with arithmetic, for example, can keep track of scores in games and can play flash card games with you. Activities for improving your child's learning skills are given in Chapter 14.

Encouragement: Special Messages to Nurture Your Child's Self-Esteem

Encouragement is the process through which a person becomes more aware of his capabilities and of his sense of belonging. Positive self-esteem develops when the child learns to feel good about what he does and about the favorable messages that others give him.

Encouragement is love. The encouraged child, the loved child, feels good about himself and about others. In giving encouragement to your child, your ultimate goal is to help him learn to apply it to himself, to accept it. Children who feel and act unloveable need the most encouragement; those who feel and act loveable receive and accept encouragement most easily. The backbone of your ability to deliver love to your child is your ability to provide encouragement for him.

Encouragement manifests itself in your underlying attitude. Your attitude is shown in many ways—by your opinions, your level of trust toward your child, your tone of voice, your actions, and the words that you say.

Encouragement is more like food than medicine; a steady diet of it over a long period of time will strengthen your child's self-esteem. It will also help prevent his self-esteem from crumbling under stress.

How to Display an Encouraging Attitude

When your child is ready to stop trying, remind him of his strength and potential. Few gifts will ever be more precious than your gift of encouragement. Here are some guidelines for establishing an encouraging atmosphere in your family:

• TALK WITH, NOT TO, YOUR CHILD. Talking *to* your child gives him no choice. It is a one-way communication in which you preach and demand unthinking obedience. You tell your child what to think, without exploring his logic. Your child receives no credit for his creativity. There is no exploring of his uniqueness, and you *insist* that your child accept your point of view. With this approach, your child soon learns to keep his feelings and thoughts to himself.

Talking *with* your child means having a two-way conversation. It shows respect for your child's uniqueness. You discover your child's logic by asking leading questions instead of preaching. Your child expresses his opinion, and you learn his point of view. You can help him correct mistaken beliefs, and he receives credit for his creativity. There is a request, not an order, that he consider your point of view. Talking *with* the child promotes harmony and is encouraging. Talking *to* the child destroys harmony and is discouraging.

• TEACH CONSTANT CHOICE. Teach your child to assert himself. He needs to learn to ask clearly for what he wants in his relations with others. Your child must not expect that others will magically know what his desires are. Ask him "What do you think you could do now?" so that he is reminded of his ability to take action to make things better for himself.

• ADJUST YOUR HELP. When you give assistance, do not give too much. There are two basic methods of adjusting the help you give your child:

1. Help is available but withheld: your assistance is offered but is not forced on your child. Sample statements include: "I will help you if you think you need it, after you've tried"; "Go ahead and try; I'll be around later"; "Do it yourself and I'll watch"; and "You know where to find me in case you need me." Sometimes a kitchen timer can be used: "Do the best you can until the timer goes off; then I'll come and see how things are going."

2. Help during part of the activity: your assistance is offered only during the beginning, or the middle, or the end of the task, but not

throughout the entire task. Sample statements include: "Would you like some help to get started? (or) at this point? (or) to finish it up?"

Adjusting your help prevents you from becoming overinvolved. Your child can feel his strength while still not being overwhelmed by fears of being left too much on his own. Adjusted help sends the clear message that you have faith in your child's abilities; giving too much help does *not* convey that message. Without physically involving yourself, you can convey your deep interest in what your child is doing.

• SHOW FAITH IN YOUR CHILD'S ABILITY. Express faith in your child's ability to cope with stresses and challenges. When you let your child undertake a task with an element of challenge or difficulty, you show your trust in him. Expect that he will be competent. The "you can do it!" philosophy is very helpful for strengthening a child's sagging self-confidence.

• HELP YOUR CHILD OVER HURDLES. Sometimes your child may get stuck at a difficult part of a task. Help him over the hurdle by giving a supportive reminder to start or to continue the activity. A statement such as "Start now and we'll see how it goes" or "All beginnings are difficult" can boost your child's courage to begin a challenging task. "How will you know you can't do it unless you try?" is another helpful statement. Focusing on the challenge and expressing enthusiasm about it can also be reassuring: "This looks like quite a challenge; it's going to be fun to see how it turns out."

• SHOW UNDERSTANDING OF YOUR CHILD'S CONCERN. A sincere expression that tells your child you know how he feels is often comforting. Statements such as: "I know this seems difficult to you" and "This is hard for you, isn't it?" let your child know that you understand his feelings. Just knowing that you do understand and care can be helpful and can often help get your child unstuck.

• EMPHASIZE YOUR CHILD'S GAINS. Point out to your child that his current performance is an improvement over past performance. For example: "Look how much your skill has improved since you first started" and "It's becoming easier for you, isn't it?"

• TEACH SATISFACTION WITH SMALL GAINS. Teach your child to notice how far he has come and to enjoy the progress that he has made. Remind him that even the longest journey starts with just a single step. Point out that mountain climbers never run up the mountain; they always take one small step at a time, and they always walk slowly. Many tasks will be beyond your child's abilities until he learns to break them down into manageable parts that he can cope with one at a time.

You can build stopping places into the task, with an instruction such as "Let me know when you have this much done; then I'll check to see how things are going for you." This method allows you to help him stay on the right track in doing the task, so that he won't have to redo parts of it. It also assures him that you will be there in case of difficulty and that you will be ready to admire his progress at each step along the way.

• SHOW CASUAL APPRECIATION OF QUALITY. Train your child away from perfectionism. Appreciate high skill, but don't put excessive emphasis on it. Although the quality of your child's performance is appreciated, it is not the primary concern. The amount of effort and degree of enjoyment that your child shows are the important aspects. Quality of performance is a secondary concern. For the highly discouraged child, it is important to comment that he has completed some of the task, without mentioning the quality level. Quality will take care of itself as long as your child is showing serious effort and enjoys the activity.

You can refer to your child's effort with statements such as: "I'm glad it's getting easier for you," and "I can see how hard you are working on this." You can put emphasis on your child's enjoyment of the task with statements such as: "It will become more enjoyable as time goes on," and "You will learn to like this as you keep trying."

• EMPHASIZE YOUR CHILD'S STRENGTHS. Say "I like the way this part was done" when commenting on your child's performance, rather than drawing attention to the errors. Trying to build self-confidence by focusing on weakness is like trying to build a house on quicksand.

Teaching Your Child to Use Mistakes Wisely

Mistakes confront your child in a never-ending parade, but they need not cause him to lower his self-esteem. They can provide an opportunity for your child to strengthen his self-esteem and to grow psychologically from his struggles to make fewer errors and achieve a greater degree of competence.

Nobody behaves perfectly. Mistakes and imperfections are a natural part of life. It is not true that mistakes must be the focus of criticism and the destroyers of your child's self-esteem. Teach your child to use them to his benefit.

It is important that you accept the imperfections in yourself and in those around you. It is also important that you handle mistakes constructively so that your child can imitate your maturity. When your child is losing self-confidence because of his mistakes, reassure him briefly by teaching him these truths:

• MISTAKES INDICATE TEMPORARY UNREADINESS. Mistakes indicate that he was not ready to do the activity. Mistakes are not proof of your child's permanent incompetence or inability to do the task. Encouraging statements are: "Mistakes sometimes mean that we aren't ready yet," or "It looks as if you weren't quite ready for that part yet."

• MISTAKES HAVE CAUSES. Mistakes are not intentional. They are excusable and justifiable. Be willing to trace the roots of the mistake. In this way, you will teach your child how to use mistakes to improve his abilities. Your child needs the courage to be imperfect, and you need to be courageous enough to allow that imperfection.

• MISTAKES ARE SOMETIMES LAUGHABLE. Look for humor and irony in situations, and laugh at your own mistakes whenever possible. This approach sets the tone for treating mistakes with the right degree of lightness. An appeal to your child to look on the bright side of his error expresses your refreshingly encouraging attitude.

• MISTAKES ARE EXPECTED. You should provide materials and procedures for helping your child bounce back from his mistakes. Build some safety nets into your activities and into your child's activities. Telling your child that there is no possibility of mistakes overemphasizes the importance of mistakes. Even though it may appear at first as though expecting mistakes is discouraging, it isn't at all discouraging when done in the proper spirit. Examples include: "That's why pencils have erasers"; "Of course there will be mistakes"; and "You only proved that you're human!"

• MISTAKES ARE ACCIDENTAL. Tell your child that you know he did not make a mistake on purpose. Treat mistakes like any other accident. They happened, they need to be corrected, and life must move on with as little wasted effort as possible. Sample statements include: "Accidents can happen, and mistakes can happen," and "I know you didn't do it on purpose."

Sometimes a child may use a mistake such as spilled milk, dropped pencils, or bumping into other children as a means of getting undue attention. In such an instance, the situation calls for discipline rather than pure encouragement. Disciplinary techniques are discussed in Chapters 12 and 13.

• MISTAKES ARE PROOF OF EFFORT. Mistakes are a necessary and natural by-product of earnest effort. The only sure guarantee for not making any mistakes is not to try to do the task at all. Remind your child that even the greatest baseball stars strike out often throughout their careers. Put the emphasis on the fact that mistakes indicate your child is trying. Avoid emphasizing the number or severity of mistakes. Examples of encouraging statements include: "Mistakes only prove you are trying," and "If you weren't making any mistakes, I wouldn't know that you were working at this task."

• MISTAKES ARE INCOMPLETIONS, NOT FAILURES. Mistakes are not reasons to stop; they are reasons to continue. Teach your child to interpret errors as unfinished work. Expect your child to continue with tasks not only until they are completed, but until they are done with reasonable accuracy. Being careful not to overemphasize quality of performance, encourage your child to correct errors in his work. A famous football coach once said after his team lost: "We didn't lose; we just ran out of time!" Your child can well use the same philosophy.

• MISTAKES ARE UNFORTUNATE BUT NOT CATASTROPHIC. The less commotion and fuss made over a mistake, the better. When your child makes errors, stay calm and quiet, give adjusted help, and be reassuring. This is sometimes hard to do, especially when your child makes the same mistake repeatedly, but patience is vital. Encouraging statements include: "The world isn't going to come to an end over this," and "Nothing is so bad that it can't be overcome." Simply reassure your child that the mistake is of little importance.

• MISTAKES ARE PROFITABLE. Teach your child that profit and improvement can come from mistakes. Challenge your child to avoid wasting the experience. Encourage him to modify his actions so that the mistake leads to improved performance. Examples of encouraging statements you might make to an older child include: "We need mistakes to show us the blind alleys so we can go back on the right course," and "The only difference between a stumbling block and a stepping stone is how you use it."

It is important not to preach at your child about how to use mistakes wisely. Instead, discuss and display your own constructive attitude toward your own mistakes. When you notice that your child is starting to be bothered by his mistakes, reassure him briefly and lovingly. By word and deed, provide a convincing demonstration of the encouraging ideas presented here about using mistakes wisely.

Chapter 6

Your Feelings About Your Child

Before and during pregnancy, both parents start to wonder what their child will be like, thinking particularly about the characteristics they would consider ideal in their baby. Such a pleasant anticipation is a normal part of preparing for parenthood. Their expectations usually include the hope that the infant will not have the faults and weaknesses of the parents and will do better in life than they did.

A baby may have special meaning for each parent. Having the baby may be the couple's attempt to pull closer to each other to save an unstable marriage. It may give the parents the satisfaction of knowing that they will soon become a family. It may symbolize masculinity to the father or femininity to the mother.

The baby is literally a product of the two parents, and if that product is defective the idealized image and meaning of the infant are shattered. The parents must cope with the disparity between their expectation of a perfect baby and the reality of a defective one. They may believe that because the baby is not perfect, they must therefore be inadequate.

Hyperactivity can exert a relentless, overwhelming stress that disrupts and harms the relationships between the hyperactive child and each other family member. This chapter focuses on these special stresses that can occur in your relations with your hyperactive child. Often the different types of difficulties have already become highly developed before the child is finally recognized as hyperactive. Even though the hyperactivity may be reduced through treatment, you might still retain some of these disturbing and potentially harmful reactions to your child. The more severe your child's hyperactivity, the more severe the stresses will be.

Early Physical Stresses

Even before the hyperactive child enters the world, resentment and fatigue may have developed in both parents. The fetus may be extremely energetic, depriving the pregnant mother of sleep by kicking all day and night. As noted earlier, some mothers have reported having their ribs bruised by their hyperactive fetuses.

Many hyperactive infants show signs of disrupted body chemistry. The baby may cry excessively and may not respond well to being held; stomach upset may occur; the baby may be unable to tolerate mother's milk; a formula that works may be hard to find. Together, these problems have been called the "failure-to-thrive syndrome." The colicky, constantly crying, unsoothable baby can quickly create a great physical and emotional stress within the family. The infant can deprive family members, and especially the mother, of sleep, quiet, and orderly routine.

What to Do: It is important that physical stresses remain just that—physical. They should not be allowed to develop into severe emotional stresses such as anger and resentment.

Mothers need rest. They have to recover from the pregnancy and childbirth as well as from the disrupted schedule and disturbed sleep that occur when the newborn infant is colicky and hyperactive. Try rotating the baby-care duties between the two parents, or get baby-care help from a relative, friend, or paid nursemaid.

Denials and Vain Hopes

As with any unexpected and threatening stress, it is often tempting to deny the existence of hyperactivity. The child's behavior can be explained away by apparently rational logic. Partly because they spend less time with the child when he is very young, fathers tend to deny hyperactivity in the child more than mothers do. The relentless nature of untreated hyperactivity, however, will eventually override the parents' denials. The denial process is usually a phase through which parents pass, rather than a permanent state in their relationship to the child.

After denial of the hyperactivity stops, another potential and tempting denial involves the belief that the hyperactivity will not be a significant stress. There may be a companion belief that it will be erased with some sort of miracle cure. There may also be a belief that after the hyperactivity is treated with medication or nutrition management, all related problems will disappear automatically. But the truth is that the effects of the hyperactivity will remain long after treatment is started. Denial of this reality is a very costly mistake for any parent to make.

Another type of denial involves the belief that a simple change in parenting technique, such as showing increased firmness or giving more loving attention to the child, will erase all of the difficulties. Such efforts by themselves, however, are ineffectual. The problem persists.

What to Do: The first step in overcoming the tendency to deny that the child is hyperactive is to realize that hyperactivity is simply a word describing a state of being. It does not mean mental retardation, brain damage, mental illness, or anything other than hyperactivity, as discussed in Chapter 1.

Recognize that hyperactivity is probably not temporary and that your child will probably not simply grow out of it. Improvement is quite possible, however, and there is much that you can do to help the child, yourself, and your family. In short, try to avoid being either optimistic or pessimistic, because both tend to blind you to the facts; instead, be somewhere in between—be realistic!

There is no final answer or solution to the effects on your family of your child's hyperactivity. There will always be some difficulties. Imperfections abound in every area of life, and hyperactivity is no exception. The steps needed to cope with it are as varied as the personalities of all of the members of your family, and no single action will solve the entire situation. Avoid a useless hunt for the perfect answer.

Attack the hyperactivity with techniques relating to body chemistry and psychology. Treatment with medication or nutrition management alone may not be sufficient. Nor is manipulation of parenting and family relationships likely to be all that is needed. Together, however, these approaches can result in very effective countering of your child's hyperactivity.

Familiarity with hyperactivity and knowledge of it are your allies, not your enemies. Every family member must understand hyperactivity. Seek professional assistance when needed, and do it without embarrassment. The hyperactivity may need to be discussed with all children in the family, including the hyperactive child. Accepting the reality of the hyperactivity means only recognizing and acknowledging its existence; it does not mean liking or enjoying it. To approach it with knowledge helps you to cope with it and gives you power in dealing with it. To deny it is to fear it and thus give it undue power over you.

Not only should you be familiar with hyperactivity, but you also must develop your abilities in parenting to an extent far beyond that of most parents. Attend parenting skills courses, discussion groups, and classes.

As your child grows, his readiness for different responsibilities, tasks, and new behaviors will change. Stay current with the course of your child's development and the changes in his limitations and his strengths.

By studying and accepting the hyperactivity rather than denying, rejecting, or minimizing it, you can lessen its power over your family.

Guilt and Inadequacy

Soon after accepting the reality of their child's hyperactivity, some parents become despairing. Guilt feelings may be especially strong if the pregnancy and birth were not well timed, or the family situation was unstable. Marital conflict or divorce during the child's early years, or any other disruption in the serenity of the family, can be grounds for the parents' feelings of inadequacy.

As time goes on, feelings such as failure, helplessness, ignorance, or self-pity can occur. All of these forms of self-hate can evolve into a bitterness about life and a defensive anger against the child.

Guilt feelings can harm many aspects of the parents' relations with the hyperactive child. Many parents tell themselves that good parents wouldn't feel the way they do and wouldn't be so resentful toward their own child. Their ambivalence toward the child, however, is not only quite normal but also quite common.

What to Do: It is natural to feel overwhelmed by such a potent force as hyperactivity. The fact that you may at times feel inadequate to the task of dealing with it says nothing about your effectiveness as a parent. Such feelings simply reflect the awesome power of hyperactivity as a stress factor on your family.

One source of feelings of inadequacy may be the failure to receive affirmation of your parenting skills from your hyperactive child. You could easily see the child who is neither obedient nor considerate as a reflection of your poor parenting. If you have at least one non-hyperactive child, notice the strengths, the cooperativeness, and the ability to give and receive love that this child has. Such traits are proof of your effectiveness as a parent. Reassure yourself by your success with the non-hyperactive child and put the cause of your child's differentness where it belongs—with the hyperactivity and not with your skills or quality as parents.

Any parent who sets perfection as a goal of parenting is inviting defeat. Work instead for improvement, and be satisfied with small gains. Perfection is useful as an ultimate goal, but it should not be the specific target of your efforts as a parent.

A common difficulty in any intense emotional relationship between two persons is a tendency to be blinded by negative feelings of anger and resentment. The positive feelings of love and caring then seem to disappear from view. Once your love bond with your hyperactive child is formed, it is permanent and indestructible, despite the growth of negative feelings. Regardless of how extreme your negative feelings may seem, you cannot completely hate any person whom you have once loved. The love bond is still there and will always be there.

This ambivalence is completely normal, especially in an intense and potentially conflict-laden relationship such as the one between you and your hyperactive child. Accepting that fact can free you from needless and excessive self-criticism. It is natural to feel resentful or angry toward the disruptions caused by your child's hyperactivity.

Overinvolvement

Parents of a hyperactive child often become overinvolved in the child's life in an attempt to compensate for their guilt feelings. There is often a great desire to run interference for the child, partly to salve the parents' consciences and partly out of a realistic concern for the child's difficulties. The parents become overworked and physically and emotionally drained from their overinvolvement, and the child becomes increasingly demanding and increasingly inept in social relationships.

Five types of overinvolvement often develop between parents and their hyperactive children:

Overprotecting

The hyperactive child's lack of caution spurs parents to become overly watchful for potential dangers. They then try excessively to shield the child from those potential dangers. The child is raised under guidelines similar to these: "Don't climb the ladder, you might fall off"; "Don't go outside without your jacket, you might catch a cold"; "Don't go swimming, you might drown"; and "Don't go for a walk, you might be attacked by dogs." The nagging fear of overprotective parents is that various misfortunes will happen to the child. In their attempt to prevent these events from occurring, the parents rob the child of opportunity to learn how to cope with difficulty or responsibility. They also reinforce their own doubts about the child's ability to cope with life. The child becomes further discouraged and convinced that his ineptness is growing worse.

A difficult stress situation for the family is hearing the many complaints that others have about their hyperactive child. The parents realize that other children blame the hyperactive child for misdeeds in the neighborhood and at school for which he is not responsible. The parents of the other children often believe their own children, adding to the pressure on the parents of the hyperactive child to be overly protective of the child. They learn to defend their child automatically, almost as a reflex.

Nagging

The hyperactive child's lack of diligence and concern for what he does can lead the parents into issuing endless directives, reminders, commands, and suggestions. The parents gradually lose trust in the child's ability to pursue his own interests or do anything independently and well. The parents become nags, and the child becomes more sloppy, slow, and forgetful and provides the parents with more to nag about.

Spoiling

Often the parents do for the child what he can and should do without assistance. Spoiling, also known as overindulging, is shielding the child from frustration by giving unnecessary and excessive attention and service. One mother summed it up clearly with this credo, which she realized she had been using as a guideline in dealing with her hyperactive child: "You just breathe; I'll do all the rest for you!"

Infantilizing

Some parents try to keep their hyperactive child in a weak, dependent, infantilized position so that they can be lavish in their nurturing.

In this way, they hope to make up for their assumed shortcomings. They may never let the child help in the kitchen, for example, so that they can take full credit for preparing all of the family's meals. The child, of course, never learns how to cook anything.

Overprotected, overindulged, nagged children do not develop constructive ways of building their strengths, and they appear and often remain ineffectual. They never have the opportunity to meet and overcome challenges in life because they have been shielded and infantilized by their parents.

Pitying

The misfortunes of a hyperactive child can remind guilt-ridden parents of their own self-assumed responsibility for having created, or worsened, the child's problems. A common mistake is to pity the child by overly sympathizing with his frustrations, hurts, or difficulties. Instead of merely showing care and concern, the overinvolved parents exaggerate the harmfulness of the child's misfortunes and convey to the child their doubts about his ability to cope. They might also allow the child to get away with little violations of medication treatment or nutrition management, which will end up only harming him more in the long run.

What to Do: Overinvolvement means taking over life experiences *for* the child rather than sharing them *with* the child. Rescuing the child from difficult situations is one example. Not involving him in solving his own difficulties teaches your hyperactive child to act even more careless and helpless the next time he is in a difficult situation and to be even more demanding of your services. Another common example is giving the child the entire solution to his difficulty instead of merely helping him to develop his own solution.

Your child may try to keep you overinvolved by telling you how awful you are if you don't do everything for him. This manipulation by guilt is very common among hyperactive children who have trained their parents to be overinvolved. You can remain strong by refusing to submit to your child's wish to make you feel guilty. Remain firm by understanding his intent without acceding to his demands.

Pity is an enemy of your child. Not only are the difficulties of life exaggerated, but your child's self-confidence is undermined. Regardless of what happens to the child, put the event in perspective and realize that things are usually not as catastrophic as we at first think them to be. It may be helpful to ask yourself: "Ten years from now, what difference will this small event make?" You will then realize how insignificant the occurrence actually is.

Your child will never learn how to swim by sitting on the shore and watching *you* swim. Only by experiencing hurt, frustration, danger, or aloneness can your child learn to cope with them. Your child will learn a lot in a difficult situation while trying hard to deal with it. The child will learn very little, however, from being rescued by you or watching you master the situation. Have confidence and faith in the child's abilities and resourcefulness, and avoid the "I can do it faster and easier" excuse for doing things for the child. Avoid doing for the child what he should be able to do for himself.

The ideal parenting style is to be concerned and involved, rather than to be *un*concerned and *un*involved on the one hand or *over*concerned and *over*involved on the other hand. When danger or difficulty occurs, reach out temporarily from the sidelines and help the child by reducing the stress in some way so that it is no longer overwhelming. Be neither an adversary nor a protector of your child.

In this way, you imply an underlying faith in your child's ability to exercise and develop his own strengths and to conduct his relationships with others.

Fears and Worries

A hyperactive child will often do some actually dangerous things, causing concern and worry for the parents. Parents worry about whether the child will hurt himself or other people; whether the child will get into more trouble; whether the child will follow through on his threats of hurting others; and so on.

Academic worries can haunt parents. If the child is promoted because of increasing physical size rather than increasing knowledge, he may never catch up academically. If the child is held back, social adjustment may be more difficult. The wide differences that the child must face in teachers' various levels of understanding of hyperactivity cause much concern for parents.

Another cluster of concerns involves the total stress that the family is experiencing because of the hyperactivity. The parents may be aware of the hurt feelings that the brothers and sisters in the family often have toward one another. The parents may be experiencing some special stress in their marital relationship in part because of the hyperactivity. At some point they may desperately consider removing the hyperactive child from the family.

Worries about what the child will be like a few years into the future are common. The child's ability to adjust to adult life may be seriously questioned, and parents may fear that the child will end up in prison or in some other sort of institution.

Additional worries occur around the question of leaving the child in the temporary care of others. Many parents cannot find anyone who is willing to watch the hyperactive child in their absence. If they find someone, they worry about the condition of their home as well as the condition of the person with whom they left the child. If they take the child with them, the child might disrupt the parents' time together. If they stay at home with the child for extended periods without a break, they may experience so much emotional stress that everyone, themselves included, will suffer as a result.

Discipline is an emotion-packed issue creating its own share of anxieties. Parents are usually concerned about setting limits, protecting others' rights, and maintaining order in the home. They may wonder how to avoid hurting the child while still providing leadership for the family.

What to Do: Bear in mind the difference between being *concerned* and being *worried.* Concern is a warm expression of interest in a potentially stressful or dangerous situation; worry is a weak, non-productive state of anxiety about the person's ability to cope with such a situation. When your child experiences your *concern,* the love bond is strengthened and an emotional bridge is being built. Your *worry* weakens the love bond and builds a wall between the two of you.

Don't just sit and stew and tell yourself that you can't do anything but nevertheless feel responsible for all of the child's problems. Do the opposite. Examine your options, take action, then free yourself of any further involvement.

Feeling Attacked and Not Understood

The parents of a hyperactive child are often confronted with an army of outsiders, each of whom has specific advice about how to solve the problems of hyperactivity. Teachers, in-laws, neighbors, friends, strangers in public places, clergymen, physicians, mental health professionals, and others often give conflicting, confusing advice. Sometimes their suggestions are valuable, but these outsiders frequently don't understand the entire situation. Sometimes they give simplistic, irrelevant advice that is based more on ignorance of hyperactivity than on knowledge of it. Parents often experience a growing sense of frustration and outrage at the inability of others to understand the true nature of their plight.

The two chastisements most often given to parents of hyperactive children are:

1. The child is not receiving enough love. The parents are scolded for not being kind or gentle enough, for not spending enough time with the child, for using too harsh a tone of voice toward the child, and so on.
2. The child is not receiving enough discipline. The parents are scolded for not being firm enough, for being too gentle, for not using enough physical punishment such as spanking, and for being inconsistent.

What to Do: It is important to realize that each of these conflicting arguments is partly true. All children, including your hyperactive child, need *both* love and discipline. For non-hyperactive children, slight adjustments in one or both of these aspects of parenting usually resolve conflicts and aid the child's personality growth and relations with others. The hyperactive child, however, may need more than just a slight adjustment. The right degrees of love and discipline are sometimes not enough to compensate for the difficulties created by hyperactivity. It is easy, however, to see how the casual or uninformed observer of a hyperactive child would quickly conclude that some adjustment in love or discipline is all that is needed.

One way to handle uninformed comments is to refuse to be surprised by them. Remember that the advice is not new, that you have heard it before, and that you will hear it dozens of times in the future. In this way, suggestions from outsiders do not become annoying irritants or big issues. They merely join a long line of similar comments which, though not helpful, are at least tolerable.

Though comments by outsiders may express blame and criticism, their underlying intent is usually to improve relations between you and your child. Try to view their remarks as a message of concern for your hyperactive child and you. Accept the spirit in which they are offered and, at the same time, feel free to ignore their critical tone. Convey your position directly to such persons by first thanking them for their concern and interest, and then proceed to respond to their specific comments.

Don't give others unnecessary power over you. Refuse to permit their remarks to harm your self-respect. Observe the principle of pleasing yourself first, rather than worrying about what everyone else will think. Accept suggestions based on knowledge, understanding, and empathy, but reject comments based on ignorance of your situation.

If you receive criticism from an outsider, explain calmly and firmly that the person is correct in recognizing that your child has difficulties, and because the child *is* special, you have obtained professional help.

In some cases, a letter can convey your feelings more effectively than a conversation. Write a detailed letter to the critical advice giver, asking for understanding and for an end to the suggestions being offered. You may also want to express appreciation for the person's concern and care in order to keep a friendly tone in the letter.

Anger and Resentment

Anger can be one of the most difficult and potentially destructive emotions within a family. It can be understood as an emotional defense against stress from outside sources, including unfairness by other people. It can be used in a controlled, manipulative fashion; people are not at the mercy of anger but are, instead, the creators of their own anger. Seething anger and resentment, which in some cases build up to tremendous proportions, are quite common among parents of hyperactive children, because of the emotional and physical stress they experience.

One source of emotional stress is coping with conflict among the children in the family. Parents may find themselves faced with the almost impossible choice of defending the hyperactive child against an angry sibling. The sibling may assert that the parents are unjust and unfair and become angry with them as well as with the hyperactive child.

Parents may discover that they cannot be alone as a couple without interruption and pressure from their hyperactive child. They may have their periods of renewal and relaxation hampered or even ruined. They may feel like his prisoners, obliged to supervise him constantly and unable to leave him alone for fear of what might happen. Over the years they may grow to resent their lack of personal space, a condition caused by the child's hyperactive behavior.

They may need to walk on eggs because the child's emotions are extreme and unpredictable. They may be embarrassed in public, hesitant to entertain visitors when the child is home, and angered because the child prevents them from presenting a good appearance to the world.

They might feel manipulated and used by the child. They may defend the child in public in a certain situation, only to discover that the child suddenly acts calm and orderly, making their concern appear foolish and excessive.

Most parents of a hyperactive child sense an invisible psychological wall or barrier between the child and all other persons, including themselves. They are aware of never having truly made contact with the child in the sense of closeness of spirit or emotional intimacy. Parents can become angry about this barrier.

Parents' anger is perhaps most easily aroused when the hyperactive child flagrantly and defiantly refuses to cooperate with their requests and rejects their leadership. They may feel a strong need to bolster their position and defend themselves against the child's rebelliousness by angrily forcing the issue.

Parental anger can be handled in many different ways. Much of it may never be expressed in direct fashion. That which is expressed directly may be aimed at the physician or counselor or teacher, at the child, or even at God with the question: "Why me?" Anger that is directed inward can turn into self-pity, self-criticism, or depression, or trigger various emotional and physical ailments.

What to Do: Don't pin the responsibility for your anger on any external source, including your hyperactive child. Your child does not make you angry, any more than someone whom you love makes you be in love with him. Instead, realize that you create your own anger, and that you do it by telling yourself certain things about what your hyperactive child does. "I'm getting angry as I listen to you talk," is a much more accurate statement than, "You are making me angry by what you are saying." Accepting the fact that the source of your anger is within you brings it within your grasp and potentially under your control.

Understand that anger is a secondary reaction to an earlier, primary emotion that involves some sort of perceived hurt or stress. Although it is possible to focus on trying to decrease your anger, it is generally more efficient to focus on decreasing the primary hurt. It is basically much easier to deal with primary hurts than with their secondary off-shoots.

Embarrassment, like anger, is reflexive; we make ourselves feel embarrassed. If you become embarrassed when your hyperactive child misbehaves in your presence in public, realize that your primary emotion is embarrassment, not anger. Then focus on taking action to prevent the embarrassment rather than trying to prevent the anger. You might, for example, remind yourself that your embarrassment is needless and perhaps excessive. Remember that it is the child and not you who is creating the scene, and that not getting upset is more important than what a handful of strangers may think about you as a parent.

Differentiate between the child and the child's behavior: the hyperactivity, not your child, is the culprit. If your child had the measles, you would be loving toward him or her and would hate to see the red spots and the other signs of the disease. You would be able to say to yourself: "I love you, and I hate your illness." In the same way, the hyperactivity can be considered the equivalent of ugly red spots which you as a parent don't like and, in fact, may learn to hate. Understand that the source of your primary hurt is the hyperactivity, not your child.

Your anger may be directed at the wall that the hyperactivity creates between you and your child. You will get angry at a wall only when you want what is on the other side. You may want to experience your child's love and the satisfaction that comes from knowing that your child senses your love for him. The hyperactivity may be preventing that form of contact. Your anger and resentment may therefore be aimed at the hyperactivity, because it blocks you from enjoyable contact with your child. Your inability to realize the full potential love bond between yourself and your hyperactive child is the primary hurt against which your anger is a defense.

Your anger may sometimes be directed at yourself for not being able to deal more effectively with your child, as much as it is toward the child. Try to become more aware of the times in which you sound as if you are angry only at your child but actually are also angry at yourself. Once you have separated the two types of anger, you can dispose of them in separate maneuvers, starting with the inward-directed anger. "I'm frustrated because I don't know what to do," is more accurate than "You are frustrating me."

Remind yourself that everyone has problems in life. There is no particular injustice in the fact that you are facing the problem of hyperactivity. Don't stop to ask fruitless questions about the justice of it all. The answer to, "How could this happen to me?" is, "Very easily, because it *is* happening!"

Lessen stresses by stopping them early. Set limits calmly and firmly. Make a clear, simple statement that the child is crossing your boundaries and that you want him to stop immediately. Back up your brief statement with a dramatic, firm, silent action that indicates your intention not to allow your child's aggravating behavior to continue. The limit-setting action should be a logical consequence or restructuring technique as described in Chapter 13.

Defending your personal boundaries *after* you are already angry is almost always a destructive process. When you feel intense anger, it may be best to cool off first, before confronting your child. Two useful techniques are screaming into a pillow as you pound it (this procedure can be done in the privacy of your bedroom), and running or walking briskly outside. When you use either method, separate yourself immediately and completely from your child. After your anger has been at least partially vented, you can then confront your child with your primary feeling, your source of hurt. You will be much more effective, humane, and strong than you would have been if you had tried to confront your child while in the midst of explosive anger. Separation from your child and removal of yourself for cooling off is not a sign of weakness or of giving in to the child; it is, in fact, a sign of your strength.

Acknowledge that hyperactivity carries with it some blessings for the child in addition to the difficulties that it creates. Perhaps your child has high energy, creativity, enthusiasm, curiosity, optimism, outgoing nature, or similar traits. Let yourself appreciate such positive aspects. In a sense, your child's hyperactivity can be viewed as a uniqueness that is not bad. It becomes destructive only when the child is in situations in which his traits work against what he should be doing. For example, there is probably nothing automatically bad about your child's need to move around a lot. When he is supposed to be sitting quietly at a school desk for several hours, however, that need becomes harmful to your child. Viewing the hyperactivity in this perspective can help you to appreciate its positive aspects.

Your child's hyperactivity is an opportunity and invitation for you to polish and refine your parenting skills. Challenges are meant to be overcome, and we grow strong in meeting them. Stimulated by the need to address yourself to the hyperactivity, you can exhibit parenting skills which can be a great gift to all of your children and a source of pride for yourself.

Emotional Bankruptcy

The parents of a hyperactive child often end up feeling completely defeated, drained, and at the end of their rope. They may have been faced with the medical stresses, feelings of guilt and inadequacy, and the emotional exhaustion of overinvolvement in efforts to save the child from impossible situations. They may have had endless worries, a flood of unanswerable questions about the child's future adjustment, and a welling up of deep-seated anger and resentment toward the child. There may have been disruption in the family, bombardment with destructive criticisms from outsiders, and a barrier between themselves and the child.

The parents may feel as if they are trying to put sixty jigsaw puzzle pieces together to make a picture that requires only fifty. Every time they make a move in one direction to get something to fit, some other situation pops up as needing their attention. Needs become stacked up against needs, so that meeting one need results in other needs going unmet. Their daily lives may become an endless struggle for peace, quiet, and calmness in themselves and in the family.

Emotional bankruptcy occurs when the parents realize that no ordinary change in parenting technique will prevent the problems that the hyperactivity creates. Treating the hyperactive child just like other children does not solve matters. Using ordinary techniques for showing love, techniques that the parents had learned to rely on with their other children, proves to be ineffectual. Relying on ordinary sources and standards for child rearing, such as the parents' friends' ways of handling their children, or what the grandparents did in raising the parents, does not work. Punishments that are dramatic and even overwhelming for other children often have no effect when applied to the hyperactive child. Spanking may bring out more intense defiance or send the child into a frenzy. There may seem to be nothing left but to yell and scream, but yelling and screaming do not solve anything. The parents end up trying everything and finding that nothing works. The parents then feel guilty because they know that yelling and constant punishment serve only to make everything worse. There may be "How many times do I have to tell you?" lectures, coupled with endless nagging. They then become as angry with themselves as with the child.

A sure sign that emotional bankruptcy has been declared is the parent's sense of defeat and the almost complete lack of any positive or loving communication between the parent and the hyperactive child. The result is that the parent runs out of options, literally gives up, and starts to feel wrung out and depressed. The parent may eventually hate to face each day as it starts. There may be a perfectionistic attempt to break the cycle, but it will be fruitless. One mother set out as a daily goal: "Today I will be calm and loving." Each day she fell short of her mark and became increasingly discouraged and depressed. The sense of hopelessness and lack of choice in the end-of-the-rope feeling is well expressed in one mother's statement: "If I'm not beating him, I'm protecting him from someone else who wants to beat him."

Feeling robbed of tools, techniques, options, and energy, the parent may conclude that there is no way out of the situation. One parent may then react by trying to dump parental responsibility onto the other parent entirely or to get the child out of the house through some social agency.

There may be a great sense of personal relief whenever the parent is separated from the child. Wholesale neglect and abandonment of the child in the home can sometimes occur. The parents may stop trying to exert any influence on the child, expressing their sense of helplessness with a "What's the use!" attitude.

A tragic reaction at this stage is child abuse. The forms of child abuse most commonly committed toward hyperactive children are: verbal abuse, emotional abuse, and physical abuse.

Verbal abuse includes excessive bossing, criticizing, swearing at the child, name-calling, use of sarcasm, threatening, insulting, belittling, yelling at the child, dwelling on the child's weaknesses and failures, comparing the child unfavorably to other children, and in other ways undermining the child's sense of worth and humanness.

Emotional abuse includes not permitting the child to feel loved. Many parents relay nonloving messages verbally. When these nonloving messages are also reinforced by acts of rejection, emotional abuse can be said to be taking place. The parent who will not do favors for the child, who avoids affectionate touching of the child, who is spiteful toward the child, who does not provide gifts for the child when gift-giving is expected within the family, who overreacts to the child's actions on some occasions while giving very little reaction to identical actions on other occasions, or who gives the child "I hate you" messages is committing emotional abuse.

Physical abuse includes hitting, slapping, strapping, kicking, hair-pulling, throwing, biting, shoving, burning, spraying, shaking, excessively twirling, excessively tickling, or excessively spanking the child. More extreme and bizarre forms of physical abuse that have been known to occur include forcing the child to eat or drink foreign substances, stabbing the child with pins, cramming objects into the child's mouth, putting the child in bath water that is too hot, and similar acts of brutality.

Not all of the actions listed here become abuse under all conditions. They become abuse when they are non-accidental, repeated, excessive in frequency or severity, and have a destructive effect on the child. For example, almost every parent feels the urge at times to spank or slap the child. When these impulses become excessive and sadistic, they constitute child abuse.

What to Do: If you are at the end of your rope, you need more than anything else to separate yourself not only from the child but also from the routine surroundings in which you relate to the child. Take a vacation; relax for a couple of days, either alone or with a friend, relative, or your spouse. You need to regain your sense of emotional balance and self-respect as well as your inner calmness and sense of personal strength.

It is much easier to *prevent* emotional bankruptcy than to get rid of it once it has started. Try to learn to surrender your need to control the child's behavior. When you have less investment in making the child act differently, the child will have less need to prove to you that you can't do it. There is only one person in the world whom you can control, and that person is yourself. Put the emphasis on controlling yourself and your own emotional reactions to the child's behavior, rather than on controlling the child. This idea is explained in Chapter 12.

Eliminating the end-of-the-rope feelings of desperation and returning to a calm and productive way of dealing with your hyperactive child is next to impossible to do by yourself. Professional assistance in unblocking your built-up feelings through counseling or psychotherapy will be a very beneficial and wise investment of your time and energy.

Chapter 7

Your Child's Effect on Your Marriage

Your marriage is the foundation of all other relationships in your family. It sets the tone for the ways in which your children will relate to each other, and your behavior helps to determine how your children relate to the two of you. Much of your impact is created by the example that you set. The ways you settle conflicts with each other, express affection toward each other, handle difficulties together, and talk with each other teach your children important lessons.

For these and other reasons, the state of your marriage must be given the highest priority. One of the greatest gifts that a child can ever receive is happily married parents.

Hyperactivity can be a dangerous threat to any marriage. It usually exerts a heavy stress in many ways. Each parent undergoes various emotional stresses in trying to deal with the child's hyperactivity. Meanwhile the two parents must continue to deal with each other. The constant change in both persons, caused in part by reactions to the child's hyperactivity, puts additional strain on the marital relationship. You and your spouse may have very different reactions to the same stress situation from your child. You will have to adjust to your spouse's reactions in addition to adjusting to your child.

As a couple, you have all of the responsibility for the usual tasks of parenting: family nest-building, homemaking, and maintaining a calm, affectionate marital relationship. In addition, you must deal with your child's hyperactivity, resolve the differences between your reactions to your child, and deal with the various stresses on any siblings.

Destructive Marital Patterns

Here are twelve of the most common marital destructive situations resulting from hyperactivity. Not all of these patterns will occur in any one marriage, and additional patterns may occur in some marriages.

Though reading this section may be discouraging or even frightening at first, it is important to be aware of the potential pitfalls which can and do happen. Many such situations evolve so slowly that the husband and wife do not realize that the patterns are developing. Few parents would admit to intentionally creating these situations in order to disrupt their own marriages, but they occur in a strikingly high proportion among parents of hyperactive children. Following this section are several steps that can be taken to help prevent or overcome these destructive marital patterns. The characteristics of many of these patterns were discussed in detail in Chapter 6.

Partial Denial

In the partial denial pattern, one spouse denies the hyperactivity while the other recognizes and correctly labels it as hyperactivity. The spouse who does not deny the hyperactivity may be criticized by the denying spouse as being too emotional or as overprotecting the child. The denying spouse clings blindly to the belief that there is nothing wrong with the child.

Joint Denial

The second parent joins the first in denying the existence of hyperactivity and then both parents are left with inadequate and self-defeating explanations for the child's bizarre behavior. Their methods of dealing with the child are likely to be equally inappropriate and destructive. Never recognizing what they are dealing with, they remain ill equipped to help the child, whose behavior becomes increasingly out of control as time goes on.

Partial Abuse

This pattern occurs when one parent becomes abusive. The other parent is not abusive and may react to the child in a variety of ways. The abusing parent may blackmail the other parent by threatening to cease all parental functions if the non-abusive parent complains about the abuse. Not wanting to assume the entire burden of raising the child, the non-abusive parent stops criticizing the abusive parent, who continues to abuse the child. Sometimes the non-abusive parent will not reveal the child's misbehavior to the abusive parent in order to protect the child from the abusive parent's temper. Other reactions of

the non-abusive parent include assuming most or all of the parental duties, becoming overinvolved with the child, and pointing out to the
abusive parent in holier-than-thou fashion: "*I* don't abuse the child the
way *you* do."

Joint Abuse

Both parents become abusive to the child in some combination of the
three types of abuse: verbal, emotional, and physical. The second parent's response to the first parent's abusiveness is to join in the abuse,
thus both justifying and denying the abuse. Couples who indulge in
child abuse usually manage to find reasons for continuing their actions.
When the abuse comes to the attention of social agencies, such couples
often move out of the geographic area rather than face the risk of losing
their children. A large number of abused children are, in fact, hyperactive.

Partial Overinvolvement

One parent becomes overinvolved with the hyperactive child. This
parent develops a habit of running interference to the point of overprotecting, spoiling, infantilizing, nagging, or pitying the child. The parent
who is not overinvolved often wants to correct the situation, and the
resulting conflict puts additional strain on the marriage. The second
parent might react in any of several ways, including overcompensating
in the opposite direction and therefore becoming somewhat abusive toward the child, or trying to one-up the overinvolved parent.

Joint Overinvolvement

Both parents become overinvolved and deal with the hyperactive
child by overprotecting, spoiling, nagging, infantilizing, or pitying.
The result is a demanding child who is unprepared to meet the challenges of life and who is catered to continually by two exhausted and
guilt-ridden parents.

Partial Emotional Bankruptcy

In this pattern, one parent declares emotional bankruptcy, forcing
the other parent to assume the total burden of parental responsibility.
In this one-sided situation, the parent with all of the burden may start
to feel angry and resentful toward the bankrupt parent and the hy-

peractive child. The bankrupt parent may feel guilty for creating such a lopsided situation but may also be quick to justify his or her actions by blaming everything on the hyperactive child with a "If it weren't for that child!" attitude.

Joint Emotional Bankruptcy

Sometimes both parents declare emotional bankruptcy. The second parent responds to the first parent's bankruptcy by joining in an attempt to unload the parental responsibility onto an external source. There may be a joint attempt to give the child away, abandon the child, or offer the child to a social agency. If the child remains in the home, there is gross physical and emotional neglect.

Another aspect of this pattern is that both parents become too dependent on outside help for advice. They gradually stop making their own decisions and thus slowly surrender their leadership function within the family.

One-Up

When the second parent criticizes the first parent, he or she eventually feels righteous and superior toward the first parent.

The first parent feels misunderstood and senses a lack of empathy from the second parent. The second parent seems not to understand the stress that the first parent is experiencing in trying to deal with the hyperactive child.

Both parents allow the primary burden of child rearing to remain with the first parent, who suffers not only from the burden of dealing with the child but also from the critical attacks of the second parent. The second parent typically claims that everything would be all right if only the first parent would change.

The second parent gains a sense of superiority by trying to label the first parent inferior, inept, uncaring, ignorant, weak, or sick. The motive for the second parent is to avoid focusing on his or her own inadequacy by keeping the spotlight on the alleged shortcomings of the first parent. Meanwhile the first parent is kept weak by the second parent's efforts to undermine any improvement the first parent tries to make.

The first parent is often overburdened. The parent who is in the one-up position is, in fact, more at ease with the child, partly because he or she is also underinvolved in the day-to-day raising of the child.

The one-up parent can announce in self-righteous fashion that he or she knows how to handle the hyperactive child and does not have so much difficulty as the first parent.

The second parent, who is in the one-up position, can destroy the first parent's efforts to improve by not showing empathy with the emotional stresses the first parent feels. The one-up parent may criticize the first parent for always wanting to prove that the child is defective. The one-up parent may also not support the first parent's attempts to learn about hyperactivity or parenting skills and may scold the first parent for seeking professional counseling. The second parent might disguise these destructive actions by claiming that the first parent ought to be able to handle the child without outside help, without taking breaks, and without trying to hunt for a label to attach to the child.

Mutual One-Up

When the first parent counterattacks after being criticized by the second parent, the two parents are then unable to negotiate mutual decisions about child rearing. They struggle for prestige and status, each attempting to feel superior to the other. Each wants to pin the blame and the responsibility for the difficulties in child rearing onto the other. Each considers the other weak, incompetent, abusive, and unfit. Both assert that everything would be all right if only the *other* parent would change. Sometimes they both will try for a one-up position in connection with something that only one of them does. If the first parent goes for professional counseling, for example, he or she may criticize the other parent for not being mature enough to accept counseling, while the other parent criticizes the first parent for being weak and needing counseling.

Sometimes the parents will weaken each other's position when one puts the other into a stress situation that he or she cannot cope with, then scoffs at the resulting incompetence and inefficiency. This pattern, if it continues and develops, can easily end in divorce.

Divided and Conquered

Primarily through lack of communication with each other, the parents can be deceived by the child's manipulations. As a result, the situation deteriorates to the point where the child needs to deal with only one parent, rather than both. The parents are thus first divided, then conquered, by the child.

The child may have become adept at using deceit to play one parent against the other. The child may find the "softy" and ask him or her for permission to do things that he knows the other parent would not allow. Another common manipulation is that the child, after being denied permission for something from the first parent, tells the second parent that the first parent has granted permission if the second parent agrees. A related manipulation is that the child, after receiving a noncommital answer from the first parent, tells the second parent that the first parent has given permission.

The child may keep pestering one parent until the parent gives in to end the harassment. Like a bulldozer, the child keeps driving forward, pushing everything, including the parent's resistance, out of his way in order to get what he wants. The child does not go from one parent to the other in this case, but bullies either parent into changing no to yes.

Hyperactive children are particularly good at bulldozing. They learn that if they nag and yell all day, the parent will be worn out and will stop fighting by evening, and they will get their way. The result is that the child resorts to bulldozing and badgering for great lengths of time, knowing that eventually the parent will wear down and surrender.

The child may bully by threatening to create an uproar. The child promises that he will torment the parents with endless pestering or throw tantrums. To the parent who likes peace and quiet, it is easier to give in to the child than to face a tantrum.

The child may also bully by threatening the parent with physical assault, by destroying property, or by hurting others. The child may defy the parent and dare him or her to use disciplinary techniques. As a power ploy, the child may goad the parent in a "Go ahead, see if I care!" fashion.

Often the child does not have to announce his blackmail weapon. The parents may already know that it exists and may apply it to themselves with little or no provocation from the child. The parents may tell themselves something like: "If I don't give in, the child will (destroy my things, scratch the paint on the car, attack his sister, steal it if I don't buy it for him, and so on)."

Sometimes the child's manipulation involves taking unfair advantage of a conflict that already exists. If the parents cannot agree on how much allowance each child should receive, for example, the child will approach the more generous parent for money. A variation of this type of manipulation occurs when the child starts fights and arguments between his parents *after* he has obtained what he wants.

Overcompensation

The excess of one parental trait in the first parent is responded to by the second parent, who develops too much of the opposite trait. The patronizing parent, for example, feels no license to be firm with the hyperactive child, because the other parent is already too harsh toward the child.

The crucial factor is not that the two parents differ in their preferred amount of softness or hardness toward the child; it is the increase in the severity of their approaches. Instead of being pulled together, the parents drive themselves farther and farther apart. The patronizing parent, for example, becomes increasingly patronizing and avoids all strictness toward the child, while the strict parent feels no license to give in to the child because the child is already being excessively given in to by the patronizing parent. Each time the child is treated softly, the firm parent will become more firm; each time the child is treated firmly, the soft parent will become more soft.

At any specific moment, the child is treated either too firmly or too harshly, depending on which of the two parents is more in control of the situation at the time. Either parent can become the too-harsh one, depending on whether dad's tools or mom's cosmetics are the targets of the child's antics.

Combinations of Patterns

These twelve destructive marital patterns can often evolve in sequence. A common sequence is the progression from emotional bankruptcy to divided and conquered. In this development, the bankrupt parent becomes the target of the hyperactive child's bulldozing manipulations and the child can then get his way with little or no resistance from the parent.

A particularly dangerous but common sequence is a progression from one-up to mutual one-up to overcompensation. Slight differences in approach toward the hyperactive child become magnified. The parents attack each other for their differing approaches. Finally they try to outdo each other by becoming more polarized and more extreme in their respective ways of dealing with the child.

Several of these twelve patterns can occur at the same time. For example, an abusive parent and his overinvolved spouse can argue about the faults of each other in mutual one-up fashion, while the hyperactive child divides and conquers them by bulldozing the overinvolved parent.

Strengthening Your Marriage

The first step in dealing with these stresses and the destructive marital patterns that can result from them is to recognize them. Spot the patterns that seem to be most likely to develop in your own marriage. Awareness opens the door to reversing these trends. Without awareness, there is no chance for an effective solution.

The greater the amount of stress in your marriage, and the more these patterns have developed, the greater the need for activities that strengthen your marriage. Regardless of how pressured or discouraging the situation is, there is always hope for improvement as long as you are aware of what is occurring.

Most of the suggestions given below apply to each parent individually as well as to the marital bond; most were discussed in detail in Chapter 6.

Hunt for the Good

Don't allow the hyperactivity to dominate your family. Search out and emphasize all of the positive aspects of your family. Help your spouse to appreciate all family members. Although your glass may seem half empty, remember that it is also half full.

Don't Expect a Perfect Solution

Realize and accept the fact that there is no perfect answer to the many difficulties that your family experiences. Part of the risk and responsibility of life is finding the best available method to adopt in any specific situation. None of the available methods will be perfect.

Seek Improvement Constantly

The more confident you are as parents, the more easily you will respond to the stresses of your child's hyperactivity. Everything you can do to increase your parental skill and knowledge will help.

In addition to improving your skill as parents, improve your skill as spouses. Study and learn as much as possible about your marital relationship. Attend workshops, seminars, classes, retreats, and similar programs that focus on marriage enrichment, and read instructive materials in this area.

Sometimes it is best to seek assistance from a mental health professional who is knowledgeable in family relationships and hyperactivity.

Defend Against Outside Criticism

One mother of a hyperactive child expressed this thought in this way: "Negative responses are like negative fields of energy—they can't do any harm if they remain grounded. I try to latch on to all the positives—friends who are understanding, a success for my child, realizing nobody is to blame when I know I have tried my hardest. If people criticize my parenting, I have begun to realize that this is *their* problem; it has nothing to do with me."

Acknowledge Your Own Role in Generating Your Anger

Talk about your self-criticisms with your spouse and urge your spouse to do the same with you. The use of anger as a weapon will decrease when you both can frankly acknowledge its self-generated nature.

Recognize Your Child's Manipulations

Notice your child's attempt to play one parent against the other. Does he bulldoze one parent? Does he find the weak spots because the two parents differ from each other about whether or not he should be allowed to do certain things? Does he hide behind the softy and push for all he can get?

Bring your child's manipulations to the forefront and deal with them as misbehavior.

Consider the events that have occurred just before you entered the situation. Before criticizing your spouse, be willing to consider an instant replay of the preceding moments. Find out what has been happening with the child and with your spouse during the last few hours.

Avoid Overinvolvement

Avoid running interference between your child and others. Let others deal directly with your child. Stand united as a couple *behind* your child, not protectively in front of your child.

Accept Differences in Approach

Accept the fact that you are both trying to do what is best for the child. Even if your approach to a particular situation is different from your spouse's, support the spouse's effort. There are usually a number of ways to handle a conflict situation, and though you may disagree, your method may not be the only effective one.

Rise above mutual criticism. Don't try to pin blame on each other. Deal with the specifics of the situation in a spirit of mutual respect and acceptance. There is nothing wrong in your spouse's being different from you, so don't attack or blame your spouse for being different. The important question in each situation is "What is the best type of parenting for the child now?" rather than "Who is the better parent?"

Switch Parental Duties

To aid your understanding of how your spouse feels, exchange roles for at least one full day. This measure is especially useful when one parent is near the point of having to declare emotional bankruptcy. The spouse can take over while the overstressed parent receives much-needed relief from the constant pressures of dealing with the hyperactive child. Switching duties is a cooperative adventure; it must never be done with resentment or as part of a one-up pattern.

Be Willing to Negotiate

Be flexible. Be willing to listen to new ideas and to the wisdom of your spouse. Remaining blindly rigid is the beginning of many destructive marital patterns. When one parent loses flexibility, the other parent may overcompensate in the opposite direction, or fall into a one-up pattern of bitter argument toward the inflexible parent. Adhering to inefficient techniques forces the other parent to go to extremes in order to start good disciplinary methods again. Sometimes these extremes are worse than the original techniques, because they create resentment between the parents. Try to come to a mutually negotiated agreement, especially in a disciplinary situation.

Use the Co-Parenting Technique

The principle of co-parenting is one of the most useful tools for preventing destructive marital patterns. Co-parenting means simply checking with each other before giving the child an answer to the child's request. The answer is a mutually agreed upon solution, developed by quick negotiation between both parents.

The negotiation should take place immediately, and it should be in private, away from the child. If you cannot arrange to discuss the matter immediately, arrange a time of day as a deadline for giving the child an answer.

Co-parenting allows both parents to balance each other in a natural, constructive way. It causes the two parental styles to come closer together; parents become less extreme, less one-sided and more flexible in coping with the total needs of the situation. The softy, for example, can help the firmer parent's point of view and can learn some reasons for being less soft and more firm. The firm parent, at the same time, can hear reasons for being less firm and more flexible.

Co-parenting protects each parent from being canceled out by the child's manipulations. The child faces two parents, not one. The parents have arrived at a unified decision through cooperation and negotiation. Playing one parent against the other in such a circumstance is impossible for the child.

Not all decisions need to be co-parented. Discuss with each other ahead of time those areas that can be decided individually by either parent. Save only the situations about which the child is likely to try to manipulate; these should be co-parented.

Arrange for Time Away

A twenty-four-hour-a-day, seven-day-a-week parent of a hyperactive child is an emotional impossibility. Allow breaks of various kinds—rest breaks, vacations, nights out of the home, and similar opportunities to relieve the intensity of the relationship between the hyperactive child and the parents. Parents who are homebound with a hyperactive child day in and day out run a risk of becoming depressed and of declaring emotional bankruptcy.

Take time for individual pursuits. Visit friends, develop a hobby, or become active in church or community work. Every person needs time alone in which to think peacefully and to enjoy a pleasant, restful activity of some sort.

A crucial type of time away is time away together. At least once each week, spend a few hours with your spouse in an enjoyable activity. Time together helps to uphold and sustain the romantic, nurturing part of your marital relationship. Unless you make sure that this special time is reserved during your weekly schedule, it can easily slip away. Nurturing activities will then be doubly needed, and your efforts will be toward making up for lost time rather than toward moving your relationship forward. Do not worry about leaving the children at home for these few hours. It is far better to have your children under the care of a sitter for a few hours each week than to have them in the hands of overstressed, overcompensating, emotionally exhausted parents who have no opportunity to strengthen their love for each other.

The importance of time away cannot be overemphasized. If you do not build in enough of it, the times when you and your spouse are together might be usurped by the practical but non-nurturing decisions that are always a part of the responsibility of leading a family.

The quality of time spent together is very important. Try to have relaxation and intimate talk, along with periods of recreational activity. If you go to a theater, talk about the program at intermission or afterward. The most crucial part of time together is the sharing of feelings in a romantic, mutually affectionate and accepting spirit. Time spent together without talking with each other is not as productive as time spent in open communication. The choice of a restaurant, for example, is not as important as the quality of the conversation while dining.

Have Regular Business Meetings

Your family pivots on your marital relationship, and your marital relationship pivots on your love for each other, which must be nurtured by romance and companionship. Having regular business meetings allows you to reserve your weekly private time together for its intended purpose—romance, not problem solving.

At regular intervals discuss with your spouse the routine problems and make the routine decisions that are a necessary part of family leadership. Decisions about time schedules, meals, shopping, home improvement, and dozens of other matters have to be made on an almost daily basis. Keep such matters in the regular business meeting, where they belong.

Give Time to Siblings

Enjoy the other children in the family. Giving them special attention to compensate for the lopsided time and energy that you both give your hyperactive child helps soothe their resentments about the stresses arising from the hyperactivity in the family. Giving them special time and attention paves the way for enlisting their help.

Enlist the Help of Siblings

Invite the other children in the family to join in helping all family members to feel confident and loved. Guide them to be alert for opportunities to compliment the hyperactive child. Ask their help in thinking of activities that they could enjoy with the hyperactive child.

Being a sibling to a hyperactive child is the world's best training ground for practicing the art of forgiveness. Use your unique family situation to guide the siblings toward accepting the imperfections of others, including the shortcomings of the hyperactive child. Urge them to build bridges, not walls, between themselves and their hyperactive sibling.

Chapter 8

Your Child's Relations
with Other Children

The emotional reactions of other children to a hyperactive child are, of course, extremely varied, depending greatly on the personality of the hyperactive child in relation to the personalities of the other children. The situation in which the children interact also influences each child's reaction to the other. There can be many positive emotional reactions to the hyperactive child: other children may enjoy his optimism, high energy level, willingness to try new approaches to tasks, or sense of humor. These positive reactions pose little or no difficulty for parents and are generally helpful to the hyperactive child's self-esteem.

Many hyperactive children, however, have a hard time establishing smooth and cooperative relations with other children. This chapter highlights the most common types of stresses that occur in the hyperactive child's relations with the children who live, study, and play with him.

The Hyperactive Child's Intrusions

Other children may sense the hyperactive child's intrusion upon their time, their activities, their personal space, and their property. Siblings often complain that the hyperactive child won't stay out of their rooms and won't leave their belongings alone. Siblings may also complain that the hyperactive child has stolen things from them or has taken things from their rooms without permission. The hyperactive child may not be reliable about returning these borrowed items, and he may be careless about the use of the objects. The hyperactive child may be accused by others of interrupting and pestering them. Siblings sometimes feel as if their time is being monopolized by the hyperactive child, and they may feel helpless to improve the situation.

What to Do: Often the hyperactive child's intrusion is an attempt to get attention from the other child. Instruct the other child in a few basic disciplinary techniques as responses to attention-getting misbehavior. For instance, have the other child leave the company of the hyperactive child when he starts being inappropriately intrusive.

A simple technique can sometimes be taught to the other child:

1. Stop whatever you are doing and look directly into the eyes of the hyperactive child;
2. Ask the hyperactive child what he wants;
3. If possible, make a deal in which you let the hyperactive child have his way, to some extent, in exchange for his no longer interrupting you;
4. End the conversation with a firm statement of exactly what you want from the hyperactive child; for example, that he not pester you.

This procedure should be used early in the interchange between the two children. This technique will gradually train the hyperactive child to ask directly and honestly for what he wants rather than misbehaving in order to have his own way.

Telling the other child to ignore the hyperactive child's intrusion is generally not a satisfactory solution. Alternatives to ignoring are discussed in Chapters 12 and 13.

Changing certain situations at home can help. Locks can be put on bedroom doors if necessary. The hyperactive child's bedroom can be located somewhat distant from a sibling's bedroom.

If violation of others' property rights by the hyperactive child becomes an issue, the most frequently taken objects can be put in secret locations or can be locked away. Arrangements can be made for the hyperactive child to earn his own belongings so that there will be no more need to borrow them from siblings. In some cases you may want to search the hyperactive child's room if there is reasonable suspicion that he has been taking other persons' things. Such a search should be done as a demonstration of your firmness in not tolerating violation of property rights within your family. This intrusion upon the hyperactive child's personal space must be done with an awareness of his right to privacy. Routine searches of the hyperactive child's room without specific evidence to justify them are more destructive than helpful.

The Hyperactive Child's Exemptions

In hundreds of subtle ways, adults treat the hyperactive child differently from the ways in which they treat his siblings, classmates, and
playmates. Often the hyperactive child gets a great deal of attention
and seems to monopolize the time and energy of adults. Other children
may become resentful and jealous of all the excitement that accom-
panies the hyperactive child. In their desire to receive equal treatment,
they may misbehave or start to imitate the hyperactive child.

Even before the adults realize what is happening, other children can
often see a pattern of overinvolvement developing. The other children
might consider the adults to be too supportive of the hyperactive child
and might become angry at their apparently biased total absorption
with the hyperactive child.

Other children may sense that the hyperactive child continually demands special exemption from rules, refuses to cooperate with established routines, and in other ways tries to claim special privileges for
himself. They may stop inviting the hyperactive child to play with
them.

One difficult form of exemption is the hyperactive child's refusal to
follow established family routines or to cooperate in doing chores. You
may have given up trying to get the hyperactive child to do a fair share
of the family's work, because all of the methods that you have tried
have failed. Though you may have resigned yourself to the uncooperative nature of your hyperactive child, the siblings may conclude that
you are extremely unfair. They may express their anger directly toward the hyperactive child or toward you, or they may refuse to do
their share of the work.

Equally destructive is the hyperactive child's tendency to violate re-
strictions, limits, and guidelines. Somehow the hyperactive child may
seem to get away with lots of misbehavior and rule violations that are
forbidden to the other children, which may result in the other children's demanding an equal right to misbehave in the same way.

What to Do: Make sure that each other child senses your unique
and special concern. Try to help the other children understand the
plight of the hyperactive child. Teach them that the exemptions are
neither as ideal nor as inviting as they seem. Jealousy will be reduced
when the other children realize that the hyperactive child's apparent

privileges come at great cost and are evidence of the hyperactive child's difficulties rather than of his success in life.

It may be helpful to point out various emotional stresses that the hyperactive child is experiencing. Assure the other children that you deeply appreciate their willingness to cooperate and their agreement not to demand similar exemptions. The other children must be able to use this appeal wisely for their own benefit. They must not repeat what you have told them to the hyperactive child to hurt him.

Helping them understand both the hyperactive child's feelings and yours allows the other children a meaningful part in the total situation. Let the other children know of your frustrations in trying to prevent the exemptions from occurring, and assure them of your desire that the hyperactive child not continue to violate routines, disobey rules, or demand further exemptions. When the other children understand that you are aware and concerned about the exemptions and that you are doing your best to keep them under control, they will be less inclined to stay angry toward you and to demand special privileges for themselves. Explain that you are aware of how difficult it must be for them to do chores or obey rules about which the hyperactive child refuses to be cooperative.

Beware of the misleading and useless admonition from your children to be consistent. One of the myths of parenting is that parents need to be consistent in every way. Actually there are several different kinds of consistency, and it is neither wise nor possible to be completely consistent at all times.

Here are some of the major kinds of parental consistency:

1. Evenness of mood, moment-to-moment and day-to-day;
2. Universality of right and wrong among the members of the family: what is unacceptable behavior in one child is also unacceptable in any other;
3. Follow-through and dependability: *all* promises and threats are kept;
4. Parents should provide whatever guidance appears to be needed by a specific child at the moment, regardless of whether a similar action would have been taken with a different child;
5. Pairing a child's actions with a certain predictable result: one child always receives the same parental response for misbehavior, but that

response may be different from that for another child for the same misbehavior.

6. Consistency in dealing with the children: all children are given the same privileges, discipline, etc. (even if the discipline may take a different form in particular instances).
7. Parental agreement and similarity of approach: the parents always back up each other when providing guidance and discipline;
8. Parental honesty and truthfulness: the parents never lie;
9. Psychological congruence: matching of inner feelings and intentions, body language, word choice, and voice characteristics with actions—the parents act in accord with how they feel.

Each of the kinds of consistency may be very desirable in certain circumstances, but in the long run some may be more crucial than others.

Sometimes a parent's single action may allow one form of consistency to occur but may prevent another form of consistency from taking place. For example, the parent may promise early in the day to treat the child to an ice cream cone after the evening meal. By the time of the evening meal the child's actions could have caused so much disruption for the parent that the parent no longer feels like doing any favors for the child. To be congruent, the parent may choose to withhold the promised ice cream cone, thereby being inconsistent with regard to keeping a promise.

The other children need to learn that while consistency is generally desirable, there are many situations in which acting consistently would create more problems than would be solved. Letting the hyperactive child get away with something may be the least destructive of the available courses of action and thus may be the best parenting technique to use. When you ask a sibling to do a chore that the hyperactive child refuses to do, you are not necessarily being unfair. Instead, you may be choosing this action because maintaining your love bond with the hyperactive child is more important than getting him to do the chore.

If you help the other children understand that you are aware of the need for consistency and are eager to apply various forms of consistency whenever they truly fit the total situation, they will be less likely to complain about the inconsistencies that remain.

Discourage demands by the other children for equal privileges. Substitute instead the concept of equally special privileges that are uniquely suited to each child. If you expect your hyperactive child's dishwashing skill to be unsatisfactory, for example, the sibling who does the dishes can be excused permanently from some other specific chore, or can be given a special privilege.

The exemptions claimed by the hyperactive child often involve routines and rules that are binding on all other persons in the class, family, or group. The other children have as much need for a safe and effective arena in which to renegotiate the rules and expectations for themselves as does the hyperactive child. Routine meetings are very helpful. Meetings can increase the children's awareness that their needs are being attended to and that their concerns about rules and routines are being heard. Hearing the concerns of others articulated in a calm forum in a spirit of negotiation is also a very helpful and humane way for the hyperactive child to gain insight into the effects of his behavior on others, and to keep his behavior in perspective. The family council method is discussed in Chapter 9.

The Hyperactive Child's Effect on the Group

Other children are often concerned about the hyperactive child's effect on the entire group, whether it be the neighborhood, the classroom, or the family.

Classmates may fear that the teacher will deprive the whole class of a privilege because of your hyperactive child's misbehavior. Playmates may fear that they will lose permission to play in certain locations or with certain children because of your hyperactive child's actions. Siblings may feel deprived of certain activities because the family's efforts to prepare for, travel to, or participate in an event are disrupted by the hyperactive child. Angered by what the hyperactive child puts Mom and Dad through, siblings may be aware of a loss of privileges and activities for the whole family because the parents are under considerable stress from the hyperactive child. They may also conclude that certain specific problems in the marital relationship of the parents have been made worse by the hyperactive child's misbehavior.

In their attempts to lessen the effect of your hyperactive child on their groups, the other children may find ways of including him only partially in their activities. They may find various ways to take advantage of him. In games such as tag, he may be "it" most of the time. If children are taking turns riding in a wagon, your child may end up doing most of the pushing. He may be assigned to less important positions in baseball, and the other children may want to quit before he gets to bat.

What to Do: Other children may sometimes be equally responsible, along with your child, for contributing to the stress of the situation. So beware of rushing too quickly to save the group from experiencing the effect of your child—they may often have had a part in keeping him upset and disruptive.

Siblings and classmates may think that your child's behavior and adults' responses to that behavior are intruding into their lives. They have a need to express those concerns in an open forum, such as the family council.

Take measures to ensure that your child's impact does not spread much beyond himself. The teacher should consider leaving behind only the hyperactive child, not the whole class, from a planned activity if the child becomes disruptive despite appropriate attempts by others to prevent the situation. Such actions may seem a bit harsh and may seem like rejection of the hyperactive child, but they are not. They should be done in the spirit of helpfulness, with explanations offered that the child is not ready to participate in the activity. Also, if others are not able to accept the hyperactive child's actions, it is better that they be honest about their feelings and avoid being with the hyperactive child. If they fail to do so, they will build up resentments toward the hyperactive child for his having ruined the event for them.

Other Children's Bewilderment

Most children will abandon actions that bring negative reactions from others. Your child's friends and siblings might therefore be bewildered at his continued misbehavior despite all of the negative feedback and reactions he incurs.

Other children may be confused about the ineffectiveness of adults in dealing with your child. They may sometimes demand that adults *force* him to behave appropriately, and wonder why he can't be stopped from doing what is obviously disruptive and inappropriate. They may fail to understand adults' frustrations in dealing with your child, and may criticize them for their apparent lack of interest in getting your child to change his actions.

What to Do: The bewilderment of other children usually stems in part from their lack of information about hyperactivity. Tell them about the nature of your child's difficulties. Help them learn not to demand that adults produce a solution to the hyperactivity in every situation.

Explain to the children that receiving negative reactions is not a good way for your child to learn. Tell them that their ability to improve their own behavior and relationships when others respond negatively is based on their having good self-esteem. Your child, however, usually does not have such positive self-esteem. Negative responses are denied and explained away, or he uses them as excuses for counterattacks, not constructively for behavior improvements. Your child interprets them as showing that he is unacceptable, unlovable, incompetent, or worthless. When they understand about his low self-esteem, the other children will not be so surprised that your child is not more pleasant to be with after receiving a constant barrage of negative reactions.

Other Children's Embarrassment

Other children in the company of your child may sometimes feel awkward and embarrassed. Classmates may suspect that the entire class is getting a reputation because of your child's actions. Older siblings may have given up trying to bring friends home to visit. The rest of the family may be hesitant about taking your child out among strangers; siblings may refuse to leave home with the family if your child is also going along.

What to Do: Separation of your child from siblings on certain occasions is one way to prevent feelings of embarrassment from developing. For example, arrange schedules so that your child is not at home when the siblings want to have their friends come for a visit. Manipulating personal schedules, however, is not a genuine or permanent way to avoid embarrassment.

A better long-term approach is to teach the other children that they create their own discomfort by developing feelings of embarrassment. Actually your child is embarrassing no one but himself. Your child, *no one else*, should be the one to experience whatever reaction his behavior receives from other people. Remind the other children that when they react to your child's inappropriate behavior by feeling embarrassed, they are allowing him to control the situation and prevent them from enjoying the event.

The other children must learn to stand aside psychologically so that they are not in the middle between your child and others who are upset by your child's behavior. Suggest to the other children that when someone makes comments to them about your child, they should ask the other person to make those comments directly to him. Other children need feel no obligation to explain, excuse, justify, apologize for, or be embarrassed by your child's behavior; the aftereffects of his behavior are his own responsibility.

Other Children's Anger

Other children often develop a great deal of hostility toward your hyperactive child because of the inconvenience, embarrassment, frustration, disruption, and even personal attacks they have experienced. Your child may have difficulty keeping friends because of a tendency to alienate other children; there may be considerable turnover in your child's friendships and acquaintances. Siblings, classmates, and playmates may openly state that they hate your child and may seem to be at war with him. They may express a desire to reject him, expel him from their groups, and in other ways dismiss him from their lives. Sometimes they may be intent on getting revenge on your child and will take advantage of almost any opportunity to do so.

What to Do: Teaching children how to deal with their anger is an important and very difficult responsibility for parents. The same lessons about handling your own anger that are described in Chapter 6 must be taught to the other children who interact with your child. They must be made aware that their anger is not directed so much at your child as at his behavior, which acts like a wall that prevents the other children from enjoying and making contact with your basically lovable hyperactive child. This idea can be clarified by pointing out to the children that harming your child would not be a right thing to do, even though there are times when your child's behavior is unpleasant. In this way they can learn to appreciate and respect the humanness and worth of the person who is behind the hyperactive behavior.

Another aspect of anger that is very important for children to understand is that it is self-generated. Point out that by allowing them-

126   FEELINGS AND RELATIONSHIPS IN YOUR FAMILY

selves to become angry they give your child undue power and influence over their lives and their happiness. Encourage them to be flexible in their needs concerning your child's behavior; it is not crucial to their survival that your child *must* change his behavior.

Stimulate the other children to think of specific ways in which they are contributing to the difficulty. Challenge each other child to ask himself: "What am *I* doing that allows the conflict to remain or grow worse?" Then challenge each child to ask the obvious next question: "What can *I change* in my behavior to help improve the situation?" The other children must understand that by asking themselves these questions, they are not defending or excusing your child's actions. Instead, they are putting their own behavior into perspective alongside your child's. In this way they learn to control their own emotional reactions toward your child and also give themselves a means of altering their own behavior to reduce the conflict.

Children who have been in stressful conflict situations with your child on frequent occasions may want to seek revenge. This need for revenge may also be found in children who have been exposed to it by adults and by their peers. The same principles described in Chapter 5 concerning your child's handling of anger also apply to helping the other children deal with their desires for revenge on him.

A dramatic, easy-to-understand demonstration of the folly and destructiveness of revenge is the following special wrist-slapping procedure. It should be used when both children are calm and not in the midst of a conflict with each other:

1. Have the two children (designated *A* and *B* here) sit facing each other;
2. Tell *A* to extend his fist with the back of the hand uppermost;
3. Tell *B* to give one hard smack to *A*'s wrist;
4. Tell *B* to extend his wrist in the same fashion;
5. Tell *A* to slap *B*'s wrist once, *harder* than *A*'s wrist was slapped;
6. Repeat the cycle three more times, each time making the slap harder than the immediately preceding one; each child receives a total of four slaps of progressively increasing sharpness.

By asking leading questions and in other ways being gentle and instructive, help both children draw the following conclusions about revenge:

1. There is no end to a revenge struggle;
2. Revenge struggles get progressively more severe and painful;
3. Revenge does not solve the basic conflict;
4. Revenge struggles hurt both people, so that there is never a winner, just two losers;
5. Revenge destroys caring and cooperative feelings; if this procedure would have continued, both children would have become very angry toward each other;
6. The person who must take definite action to end a revenge struggle is the last one attacked, not the one who strikes the last blow;
7. Revenge struggles are silly and pointless.

Once they have performed and discussed this procedure, the children will not forget it. Use it to remind them to avoid revenge struggles with the hyperactive child. Whenever you notice that they are acting revengeful, challenge them gently with a question such as, "Are you trying to play that wrist-slapping game again?"

Rivalry

Other children often become highly competitive toward a hyperactive child. Sometimes they may be jealous of the special attention your child receives. They might be angry and resentful about your child's intrusions or negative effects on the group. Your child may display a boastful, "I'm the best" attitude, which invites an answer. The desire to compete with your child may be coupled with a desire to dominate or defeat and thus, symbolically at least, to destroy him. This intense competitiveness, while perhaps tolerable in a play group, is definitely undesirable in a classroom and destructive in a family.

What to Do: Help the children understand that cooperation, compromise, and sharing are desirable and are supported by adults. Likewise, make it clear that competitiveness is basically not supported. Urge the other children to compliment and share with your child, and encourage him to do the same.

Emphasize your separate and unique love for each of your other children as well as for your hyperactive child. Children are different from one another and both parents must show a different kind of love for each child.

Children tend to compete for their parents' attention when they fear that there is not enough love in the family to go around. They can be reassured by talking with them about their love for their pets. Point out that each pet is unique and has its own special traits but that each pet is loved by the family. The fact that the child loves one pet does not mean that he or she has less love for the other pet. In the same way, the parents' love for one child does not detract from their ability to love another, or mean that they will love their other children less.

Avoid the mistake of trying to keep everything absolutely equal among all of the children in the family. When a big point is made about each child's receiving no more and no less than any other child at any time, the children tend to become very jealous and demanding. Give different gifts or privileges to each child, based on his or her uniqueness and readiness as well as your own needs. When each child realizes that he or she will get different and special things, there will be no demand that you owe identical privileges, attention, or gifts every time the hyperactive child gets them.

Sometimes you may be tempted to help the hyperactive child by urging him to do as well as an older brother or sister in some activity or skill. Direct comparisons, however, are insulting and discouraging. The child who already shows the desired behavior may be eager to maintain the favored status and may try to prevent any progress that could be made by the hyperactive child. Or he or she may fear that it will be difficult or impossible to continue to meet such high expectations and may become discouraged. The hyperactive child will certainly be discouraged, because his inferiority has just been emphasized.

By showing a separate and unique love for each child, by avoiding a concern for complete sameness and equality in gifts and privileges, by spending regular time alone with each child, by avoiding direct comparisons, and by encouraging compromise and sharing, you can help your other child or children develop consideration and a helpful, noncompetitive attitude toward the hyperactive child.

Chapter 9

Rebuilding Family Harmony

Love and discipline are the twin bases for effective leadership and harmony in the family. If there is too much or too little for each child, the relationships in the family become strained and children's misbehavior increases.

Of the two, love is the primary, the basic need. It is the rock upon which sound discipline must rest. Without love, discipline can be unauthentic and uncontrolled to the point of child abuse. The most successful method of restoring harmony in your family is to provide judicious discipline as well as genuine love to all of the children. The effective parent is very firm *and* very loving.

Rebuilding Family Harmony through Increased Love

As your child's behavior changes and improves, your approach must also change. Improvements must be acknowledged and appreciated, and parents, relatives, teachers, and friends must welcome this progress. Discontinuing your old habits and responses are important aspects of adjusting the love and the discipline you give your family. As your child responds to your increasingly effective disciplinary approaches, harshness or anger that formerly may have seemed necessary will become excessive. There will be fewer moments in which a raised voice or an angry look will be appropriate. When you receive a negative report about your child, give yourself time to analyze the complaint. Control your reaction, and avoid taking sides if possible.

The expectation that the hyperactive child will be the main source of irritation in most conflict situations is a difficult habit to break. As the child's behavior becomes the true cause of difficulty less frequently, you will be able to see more clearly the roles of others, particularly brothers and sisters, in directing adults' anger. The habit of expecting the child to oppose you whenever you ask him to do something may also be difficult to stop.

The temptation to go on witchhunts, the reliance on punishments as solutions to conflict, the tendency to nag and scold repeatedly, the desire to ignore the child's behavior, and the parental tantrums are all responses that must be toned down and eventually eliminated. These inefficient methods of discipline, discussed in Chapter 12, will slow the progress of your child's improvement.

Introducing more love into the family will be much easier if both parents share this goal. Any improvement in the marital relationship will, of course, promote an increased feeling of love and harmony throughout the entire family. This important facet of rebuilding family love was discussed in Chapter 7.

Find occasions to thank your children for doing things. Too often, children hear about the things that they *don't* do, or don't do correctly. Even little acts like bringing in the newspaper or the milk can be noticed and appreciated. Doing small favors provides ways for everyone in the family to show their love for each other on a daily basis.

Make every holiday into a chance for the entire family to join in the fun and to enjoy each other. Show family movies and slides often, and assemble picture albums and family scrapbooks. Have pictures of family members on the walls of your home. Be alert for opportunities to give all family members a greater sense of unity and togetherness.

The following activities will also help to promote harmony in your family by increasing everyone's sense of being loved:

Family Cooperative Ventures

Work and play together as a family unit with the common goal of cooperation and companionship. Anything from cleaning house to building a sand castle together can sustain and enhance the family's love for each other. Focus on the positive aspects and not on the shortcomings of the activity. The project should involve something that the entire family will use. Examples include having a family garden, pitching a tent, painting a trailer or a boat, setting up a model train layout or doing home remodeling.

Talks About Feelings

Have family conversations in which members take turns talking about gaining new insights, avoiding self-defeating behavior, being fulfilled, being excited, having a success experience, or similar good feelings.

Thanks to Each Other

Expressions of gratitude sustain love. The family can sit together, with each member expressing thanks for something that another family member has done recently. The gratitude can be on behalf of someone else, so that the person expressing thanks need not be the person who was directly benefitted by the person being thanked. Each member of the family can be asked to tell at least one other family member the circumstances in which he or she appreciates the other family member the most. Another idea is to have a thanks-sharing circle, in which the family sits in a circle and each person gives a sincere message of gratitude to the person next to him. Variations on this theme are endless. One family has a love message center consisting of large envelopes with pockets. Family members write notes of appreciation to each other and deposit them in the envelopes; the messages can then be read privately or shared with the family once a week.

Gift Exchanges

Some parents have not learned to be comfortable about accepting gifts from their children. Too often parents reject offerings from their children or dismiss the gifts as unimportant. Gift exchanges usually work best if family members exchange gifts with each other. Gifts can be tangible or can involve service or activity such as playing a game, giving a back rub, or doing a favor. The custom of giving gifts on holidays is a form of love-gift exchange.

Special Days

Give each family member a day to be "king" or "queen" and to do just about anything, including being free of the usual responsibilities and obligations. On the child's Special Day, he or she can have a special table setting to eat from, wear a special hat, have favorite meals, and choose family fun activities for that evening. Special days can be given whenever something out of the ordinary is happening for the child, such as a birthday, a job particularly well done, or the first or last day of school. They can also be arranged for fun reasons, such as unbirthday, half-birthday (six months from birthday), kindness shown to others, or just because.

Family Togetherness Times

Arrange regular times during which the entire family gets together for work, discussion, or play. Put all other matters aside so that every family member can give full attention and involvement to the family activity.

Parent-Child Pairing Times

Each parent should spend some time alone with each child, devoting his or her full attention to that child in an activity that the child enjoys. The child basks in the full and undiluted love and attention of the parent. These times provide good opportunities for closeness to develop between parent and child, especially for the parent who is uncomfortable at showing affection in front of other family members.

Family times and parent-child pairing times need not involve games on every occasion. Simple companionship activities that are enjoyed by all participants can enrich the family's love for each other. Reading stories, playing with toys, exercising, taking a walk together, and similar activities will all prove useful for this purpose. Whatever the activity, it is important that parents and children come away from it enriched and renewed in their love for each other.

Surprise Times

Notes that describe pleasant surprises can be included in each child's lunch box or given in some other way once each week. The surprises can include favors and privileges, such as lunch in a restaurant of the child's choice. Surprises should not be coordinated strictly with the children's behavior; they are more effective if given for no particular reason as an indication of constant love for the children.

Rebuilding Family Harmony through Cooperative Play

One of the principal ways to increase love in the family is to have a regular playtime, which can involve parent-child pairs or the entire family. A regular playtime has several advantages for the parents as well as for the children, as discussed in Chapter 14.

Play is an activity through which learning takes place, and among the things learned in play are attitudes toward interpersonal relationships. Cooperative family activities are important aspects of your family's relationships, and cooperative games can be a great help in rebuilding harmony in your family.

Self-love and love of others cannot blossom in a competitive atmosphere but can flourish in an atmosphere of cooperation and mutual respect.

Cooperative games differ from competitive games in that the factor of persons being pitted against each other is minimized or absent. If the play activity is bitterly competitive, some unfortunate attitudes may be learned by the winners as well as by the losers. Instead of a winner who defeats a loser, all players work toward a common goal. All players win if the goal is reached and all lose if the goal is not reached. The other uncertainties and obstacles of games, such as skill and chance, remain.

Sometimes the goal is that all players finish their parts of the game at the same time. In cooperative Chinese Checkers, for example, all players try to place their last marbles into home place on the same round. In cooperative regular checkers, the players try to change the black and red checkers to opposite sides of the board at the same time with no jumping or moving backward.

All players can try to coordinate their timing and actions with other players so that a smooth pattern of action develops. In cooperative ring toss, for example, one player holds a stick and tries to catch rings which are thrown toward the stick by the other player.

Players can take turns, one after another, in reaching the final goal. In cooperative jacks the first player picks up one jack, the second picks up two, and so forth, until the goal of a certain number of jacks is reached.

In cooperative sentence writing, the players take turns adding a new word to the sentence. Players do not communicate with each other about what the sentences will say. Any player can add punctuation in addition to a word during his turn. The sentences that result can be read aloud for everyone's enjoyment. In cooperative picture drawing, each person makes a stroke with a pencil or crayon (or chalk on a chalkboard) during his turn. Each player adds a little bit to the drawing during each turn, with no communication between players. The picture evolves naturally from the cooperative spirit and creativity of the players.

Sometimes a total score for the entire group can be agreed upon before the game starts. In four-player card games there are thirteen possible tricks. Before any player sees his own hand, the number of tricks he must take should be agreed upon. Players can then cooperate in trying to help each other take the correct number of tricks.

With no other teams or players to compete against, players can agree on modifications of the game as it progresses. This flexibility provides more creativity and more variations; new games result. More planning takes place while the game goes on, and the entire experience becomes a more fulfilling activity than an ordinary competitive game.

There is less resentment toward any one player's errors or inefficiencies in performance. For children who have coordination problems, this aspect of cooperative games makes them especially helpful. The group as a whole often attempts to compensate for errors made by any one player. Fewer quarrels break out; children seldom accuse each other of cheating, lying, not knowing how to play, being afraid, being weak, being poor losers, or being show-offs. Any one person's outstanding abilities become assets to the entire group rather than becoming obstacles to opponents.

Storytelling can also be a delightful family activity. The children can take turns acting out the story being told, or they can take turns adding segments to the story.

Those times in which the entire family is together in a car also provide opportunity for cooperative family fun. Many varieties of word games and guessing games can be used, in addition to such cooperative activities as singing and joke telling.

In many cooperative activities, coordination, timing, and rhythmic movement are involved, so that a pattern of motion and momentum develops. Cooperative games are generally enjoyable from a physical standpoint as well as from a psychological one.

Rebuilding Family Harmony through the Family Council

The family council is one of your most powerful tools for rebuilding and maintaining a new level of harmony in your family. The basic idea is simple: regular meetings of the entire family to discuss issues, make plans, voice concerns, solve problems, agree on solutions, and celebrate your love for one another. The family council is essentially a method of allowing your children a voice in the affairs of the family while at the same time providing you with an avenue for exercising your leadership in a benevolent way.

A typical family council meeting has a schedule similar to this one:

- REVIEW OF LAST WEEK'S ACTIVITIES. The pleasant activities of individuals and of the whole family during the preceding week are discussed, to refresh memories and to bring everyone up to date.

- NOTES FROM LAST MEETING. Notes from the preceding meeting are read aloud. They include the issues that were discussed as well as the agreements, decisions, and plans that were made.

- PERSONAL SCHEDULES FOR THE UPCOMING WEEK. Transportation, child care, meals, and similar routines may need to be modified for one or more family members during the upcoming week. Any deviation from routine schedules is announced, so that all members know where everyone is going and, in general, what everyone is doing.

- FAMILY PROJECTS FOR THE UPCOMING WEEK. A discussion takes place about recreational and family fun activity as well as family work projects. Decisions about how the family will spend the upcoming weekend, for example, occur during this discussion.

- CHORES AND ROUTINES. Any family member can make suggestions for changing the routines which are necessary to keep the family functioning. Discussion includes such items as clothing, meals, housework, lawn care, pet care, car care, and room cleaning. Discussions take place about whether previous decisions have been carried out, and if not, why not.

- CONCERNS AND NEGOTIATIONS. Items dealing with long-range family plans, such as vacation planning, job changes, residence relocation, or household remodeling are discussed. Any difficulties or conflicts that any family member is experiencing can be discussed. Various solutions are proposed, and agreement is reached on which solution to try, usually for an experimental period of one week until the next family council meeting. Because the hyperactive child may have difficulty maintaining well-controlled behavior for long periods of time, he has a greater chance of being successful if he has an entire week for trying new behavior.

• RECORDING OF AGREEMENTS. One person takes on the secretarial duty of reviewing and recording the agreements and the plans made during the meeting. This record helps to prevent future misunderstandings among family members. It can be written or tape-recorded.

• LESSON. A lesson is taught to the family by one or two family members. The lesson can involve religious, moral, or social values and may include visual aids or other entertaining features. Usually the lesson consists of a presentation followed by discussion which involves all family members.

• ALLOWANCE. Financial matters are discussed, and allowances are distributed to the children.

• CELEBRATION. The council meeting closes with games, singing, storytelling, refreshments, or some similar celebration of family life. Celebrations can be rotated, so that each week a different child is responsible for providing the fun activity or the refreshment. With a little bit of advance planning, the celebration can become a basis for regular parent-child togetherness for the purpose of preparing and cooking the refreshments.

Among the important parental leadership functions in the family council meeting is the guarding of each person's right to express genuine concerns and opinions. In this way the children learn that they can have impact on the family's decisions. As the children learn that their opinions are valued and listened to, they will gradually put more thought into them. More and more useful suggestions will be offered as time goes on.

As each issue is discussed during the family council meeting, each family member needs to examine it from the viewpoint of the needs of the entire family.

The decisions in the family council meetings are agreements; they are made unanimously or by consensus, with each family member participating. Consensus differs from majority rule, which is not agreement at all. Agreement is not reached until all family members, not just the majority of them, can endorse and be comfortable with the proposed solution or plan of action. In majority rule, of course, those who disagree are outvoted.

In order to attain consensus, a thorough search must be conducted of all of the facts. Everyone's opinion must be considered, and the ideas which meet the needs of most family members should be offered as temporary solutions, at least until the next family council meeting. If no agreement can be reached, decisions are postponed until the next family council meeting.

The most important attitude is a spirit of inquiry. Guiding questions include these: What is the situation? How does it look to each family member? What ideas can be proposed to improve it? Which one holds the most promise? What shall we do to make sure that it is tried? Inquiry and discussion are done in the spirit of mutual respect for everyone's viewpoint and everyone's right to make choices.

The most common abuse of the family council meeting is to treat it as an opportunity to lecture to a captive audience. If you use these meetings to preach, scold, or impose your will on your children, they will fail in their purpose. One way to help ensure a high level of openness of communication is to rotate the positions of chairperson, secretary, and lesson giver so that the children gain a sense of participation and responsibility.

The family council meeting must not be allowed to deteriorate into a gripe session. Each person expressing a complaint is also expected, if possible, to present one or more suggested solutions at the same time. The emphasis is not on how any *one* member should change, but on what *the family* can do to prevent a certain difficulty from arising in the future.

An additional function of parental leadership at the family council meeting is to make those decisions which are parent-level decisions. Deciding whether the family needs to relocate and if so, where, for example, is essentially the parents' decision. The family council meeting is an excellent arena, however, in which to find out the children's feelings about the upcoming move, and to receive their suggestions for making the move more pleasant for the family.

The first few family council meetings should be oriented toward making plans for pleasant activities, such as deciding about weekend projects or vacations. In this way, the family can become accustomed to the concept of regular meetings without having to face difficult or touchy negotiations. Other parts of the typical family council meeting can be included later, as the members gain increased practice, confidence, and trust in each other.

It is helpful to provide a notebook or bulletin board on which family members can write the concerns and issues that they wish to discuss at the upcoming family council meeting. In this manner, all conflicts can be brought before the family, analyzed, and used as teaching examples. All members can then learn how to prevent or reduce such conflicts and how to build and maintain harmony. Gradually the family council meetings will reduce contention among family members.

Sometimes a child may feel so out of place and unwelcome that he shuns participation. Also, some children boycott the family council as a way of displaying their power or as an attempt to hurt the rest of the family (see Chapter 12). All members are invited to participate, but attendance should be voluntary. The best way to lure an uncooperative family member into participation is to conduct effective meetings over a period of time. Eventually the member will participate, out of curiosity if for no other reason.

Even preschoolers can participate to some degree in family council meetings. Certainly the younger children can help prepare or serve the refreshments. With the aid of a tape recorder, a nonreader can serve as secretary for the meeting. Whatever their role or contribution, young children can be encouraged and helped by parents to express themselves during the meeting.

YOUR CHILD AT SCHOOL

Your child's school experiences provide many opportunities for improving social and academic functioning as well as self-esteem. Unfortunately they also provide many chances for personal discouragement, resulting in great social and emotional damage.

The reality of your child's school situation may be shockingly inferior to the description given in these chapters. Many schools have great difficulty dealing with hyperactive children. Often the children spend many hours in the principal's office. Resource teachers often are not trained to meet the academic needs of hyperactive children. Teachers in regular classrooms usually have a number of students with learning or behavior difficulties and may lack the time, training, or interest to give a hyperactive child the necessary attention. Other resource persons, such as school psychologists and counselors, are usually occupied with the concerns of hundreds of students and may not be able to be of much help. There is no avoiding the fact that the hyperactive child often has a difficult time at school.

The approaches that are most likely to be of genuine help to your child will be discussed in this section. The ideal school and teacher are fictional in that no individual school or teacher has ever shown *all* of the constructive traits described in these chapters. The ideal, however, is the direction in which to head.

Be willing to show these two chapters to your child's teachers and other school personnel. Encourage teachers to move toward the approaches given here. Don't assume that they are already using them.

Chapter 10 deals specifically with gaining the good will and cooperation of school personnel, and Chapter 11 outlines teaching strategies which have proven to be most appropriate for hyperactive children.

Chapter 10

Getting Help at School

Special care for the hyperactive child in schools ranges from elaborate special classes to no help of any kind. The extent of awareness and cooperativeness among teachers and principals is very wide. At one extreme there is flexible willingness to engineer individual approaches; at the other, outright denial that hyperactivity has ever existed in any child!

Public law 94-142 provides legal assurance that educators will meet your child's educational needs. Requirements stated in this law include an individualized educational program for your child, assessment of your child's academic strengths and weaknesses, and various types of meetings and working relationships with you. This law is of great help to all parents of hyperactive, learning-disabled children.

Your Role

Aided by the existence of public law 94-142, you can insist that your child's school follow through with the development of a suitable educational experience. Several types of actions by parents have proven useful for obtaining better educational services for hyperactive children.

Obtaining an Academic Evaluation

The appropriate academic diagnosis will determine:

1. your child's present knowledge level, including areas of strength and weakness;
2. whether there is a discrepancy between what your child is learning (achievement) and what your child is able to learn (capacity);
3. the processes by which your child receives, stores, and expresses information in the classroom;

4. your child's method of attacking academic tasks;
5. whether your child has a learning disability;
6. your child's behavior traits which are most likely to interfere with participation in the classroom.

Although it usually will not include all of these areas, the testing specialist's initial evaluation may include measurement of muscle coordination, intelligence, knowledge level, reading skill, visual perception, auditory perception, language functions, speech functions, memory, emotional status, and behavior patterns in the classroom.

The initial evaluation should include a visual examination that goes beyond the simple check for color blindness. Vision problems can create a state similar to hyperactivity, which includes restlessness, irritability, and difficulty in paying attention in class. Detailed visual examination, of course, should be left to medical specialists.

Speech evaluation should include your child's ability to pronounce sounds expected at his age level, to produce combinations of sounds in certain sequences, and to express ideas with well-chosen words. It should also include a hearing check. Evaluation by a speech therapist should be done if indicated by the teacher's observations in the classroom.

A reading evaluation should be done if there are any indications of reading difficulty. Reading is a crucial skill, and difficulty in reading leads to patterns of failure among schoolchildren. Fortunately, schools usually emphasize reading skills in the early grades.

The results of the academic evaluation should be discussed and explained to you. They should be put to proper use by the teacher and by supporting personnel within the school. Unfortunately, some teachers welcome diagnostic evaluations because test results give them an excuse for their failure to succeed with the child in the classroom. Obviously, instead of being used in such a way, the results of the academic evaluation should guide the teacher toward adopting techniques that will be most helpful to your child.

Securing the Teacher's Cooperation

Cooperation between home and school is essential. It is important that you not be too soft. Maintaining an apologetic I'm-sure-you-know-best attitude toward the teacher is like handing a signed blank check to a stranger. State clearly and strongly what you expect the school to do for your child, and be sure expectation is understood, rather than a vague wish. Sitting quietly and suffering in silence while the school personnel overlook your child's academic needs is not the way to get help. To allow this lack of attention to occur is to permit the school personnel to violate their obligations to you and to your child, as well as the law. The school personnel will respect you and be more cooperative if you are polite, self-assured, and firm in expressing your expectations while at the same time making clear your intention to assist them in any way possible.

Do not assume that the teacher is an expert on hyperactivity or learning disabilities. As your contact with the teacher increases, you will be better able to gauge his or her skill and knowledge about your child's academic and emotional needs.

The local chapter of the Association for Children with Learning Disabilities (ACLD) may be of significant help in bringing your concerns to the attention of responsible school authorities. Joining a local ACLD chapter, or organizing one if none exists in your community, is a wise step. (A complete list of ACLD state affiliates appears in the Appendices.)

Sometimes a well-meaning teacher will not recognize your child as being hyperactive or as having learning disabilities, even though there may be definite problems with the child in the classroom. The teacher may describe symptoms without realizing that they constitute a hyperactive condition. During a conference, for example, the teacher may say that your child would get along better if he would sit still longer, write more legibly, slow down and take his time, not talk so much, or not hit the other children.

Even though the teacher may be able to recognize hyperactivity in general, he or she has never had *your* child in class before. Suggest the types of activities in which your child functions best, and request that these activities be included in the classroom as often as possible. Tell the teacher which disciplinary techniques work best with your child. Discuss your child's hobbies, interests, and activities. Give pertinent information about your family and the child's personal history.

Being careful not to offend, suggest that the teacher read this book, so that the two of you will have a common ground, a shared understanding, from which to coordinate your efforts. Many teachers who would not be ready to accept instruction from parents would accept it from authoritative written sources. Remember that the goal is to see that the teacher becomes informed about hyperactivity in general and about your child in particular.

Sometimes the school's inservice training programs can include discussion of hyperactivity. In many school districts, topics for inservice training come from parents' suggestions. It may be possible to get in touch with the person who is responsible for developing inservice training within your child's school and to present that person with a list of possible speakers on the topic of hyperactivity.

Urge your child to develop an open, frank relationship with his teacher and to discuss with him or her any problems that he is having at school. Send your child to school after a good breakfast each morning, so that he will not be tired as he starts the school day. These actions will communicate to the teacher your desire to maintain an effective working relationship.

Overcoming Harmful Attitudes

The majority of teachers and principals are aware of hyperactivity and are sensitive to most of the special needs of hyperactive children. The minority who do not deal realistically with the issue of hyperactivity have various ways of hindering your child's opportunity and right to assistance.

Some of the most common excuses and justifications teachers use for not meeting a hyperactive child's educational needs are these:

• SELF-RIGHTEOUSNESS. The teacher claims to believe in a desirable general principle, in a tone that assumes the parents do not share the same view. For example: "I believe that children should be able to learn in a classroom," "I believe in well-behaved students," and "I believe that students should cooperate with their teachers."

• OVERBURDENING. The teacher claims to be overworked and is quick to point out many other duties and responsibilities. For example: "I have thirty other students," "I am on several committees," and "I'm too busy with other projects to spend a lot of time with your child."

• NO TIME. The teacher claims to have insufficient time in which to diagnose and help your child's academic weaknesses. For example:

"There are only forty-five minutes in a class period," "We have too much to cover in the class," and "I don't have enough time to meet the needs of even the successful students, let alone the unsuccessful ones."

• PASSING THE BUCK. The teacher asks you to talk to a second-line helper about your child. For example: "If you don't like what I'm doing, talk to the principal," "Talk to the counselor about your child," and "The psychologist didn't give me the report on your child."

• INADEQUATE SUPPLIES. The teacher blames his or her lack of interest in your child on inadequate equipment, materials, or facilities. For example: "The book is written at too high a level for your child," "All of our materials are at too great a level of difficulty for your child," and "I could help him if I had him in a different class."

• NO EXCEPTIONS. The teacher denies that your child warrants any sort of special attention. For example: "I'm not going to kowtow to your child," and "If your child can't get along in my class, he should get out."

• RIGID STANDARDS. The teacher will not seek permission to alter grading methods or criteria to accommodate to your child's weaknesses. For example, "There is no excuse for your child's poor work," "If I make an exception for one, I have to make it for all," and "I don't want to water down my course."

• IGNORANCE. The teacher claims to be overwhelmed by your child's special needs. For example, "I haven't had the training for dealing with this type of student," "I've never developed such a program before," and "I've never had a child like yours before."

• LIMITED CONTACT. The teacher points out that he or she will not be seeing your child for a significant period of time. For example, "Why should I develop special methods when he'll be leaving in nine weeks?" and "I would not be able to help him very much anyway."

• PERSONALITY CLASH. The teacher claims to have traits that conflict with those of your child. For example, "I just can't work with your child because we're too much alike," "I just can't work with him because we're too different," and "I really don't have the patience to work with your child."

• BLAMING THE CHILD. The teacher blames the child for his lack of academic success. For example, "Your child was tardy too often . . . sulks all period . . . visits with his friends too much . . . keeps tearing up his papers . . . never does his work . . . doesn't really care whether he does a good job . . . is always seeing the counselor . . . is always hunting for excuses to get out of work . . . won't pay attention."

• BLAMING THE PARENT. The teacher blames you for preventing academic success. For example, "You just undo all of the progress that I could make with your child," "What your child needs is more discipline at home," and "What your child needs is more love at home."

Of course there are circumstances in which each of these excuses has some validity. If the excuse is true, then a conflict exists which needs to be resolved before educational progress can be made. If the excuse is merely the teacher's attempt to sidestep the obligation to deal appropriately with your child's special needs, then an even more severe conflict exists.

Some teachers like the challenge of meeting special educational needs of their students, and others don't. If the teacher clings to any of these excuses for your child's lack of progress, you may want to risk a confrontation. State in a matter-of-fact tone that it seems your child is posing some difficult problems for the teacher and that no matter what is tried, the teacher finds fault with the solution. Try to maintain a reasonable, cooperative position during this conversation. Disarm the teacher by displaying empathy and understanding of his or her frustrations.

In maintaining the delicate balance between your firmness and your understanding of the teacher's frustrations, show an awareness of the rights of the other students in your child's class. Teachers generally become antagonistic toward parents who selfishly try to manipulate classroom techniques to their own children's advantage at the expense of the other children.

In time, the teacher may be able to acknowledge that the excuses he or she offered are not valid. Perhaps over a period of several weeks the teacher may show appreciation for your understanding that he or she feels overwhelmed by the task of meeting your child's academic needs. From that point on you will find the teacher to be an understanding ally, because now both of you have experienced similar feelings in relation to your hyperactive child.

If needless delays and excuse-giving by school personnel occur, don't remain silent about them. Talk to the principal or to school board members about getting a better program and special resources not only for your child but for other children with similar difficulties. Be prepared, however, for an uphill struggle. The school officials may ask you to form a parents' group or work on some committees, secretly hoping that the busywork will get you off their backs and will satisfy your need to feel important. If you do become engaged in these activities, make your presence known and continue your advocacy for reform within the classrooms.

Do not automatically interpret hesitancy on the teacher's part as an effort to avoid helping your child. The vast majority of teachers are willing to do all they can. If you approach the school and the teacher as an adversary, you will find them to be adversaries in turn. If you approach the school personnel as potential allies, you will usually find them to be a cooperative team.

Maintaining Contact with the Teacher

Communication between you and the teacher will usually occur by one of five methods: school visits by you; home visits by the teacher; conferences; telephone; and notes. Each method has its strengths and weaknesses.

• SCHOOL VISITS. Sometimes you may be able to volunteer to work at the school as an aide. This arrangement may help the teacher by providing time for him or her to give your child the special attention that he needs. It also keeps your child on the teacher's mind and makes it less likely that the teacher will be unfair or lax in meeting his or her obligations toward your child. Depending on the circumstances, you may or may not want to serve as an aide in your child's classroom. Vis-

iting the classroom to observe your child, without actually volun-
teering your services to the school, is another type of school visit that
may be beneficial.

• HOME VISITS. Seeing your family in its home setting can provide the
teacher with a better understanding of your child, especially if he behaves much differently at home than at school. It may be helpful for
the teacher to gain a new perspective toward your child by seeing how
he acts in a different setting.

• CONFERENCES. Conferences are very important. They provide a
chance for you and the teacher to examine your roles in helping your
child. Each conference should be prearranged and should be prepared
for by all persons involved. The teacher's preparation should include a
review of your child's past academic work, recent summaries of his attitude and behavior, and examples of current work.

Your preparation should include checking to see that you have received all report cards for the current year; that you have a copy of the
school's current handbook dealing with suspension, promotion, attendance, special educational programs, and similar information; that you
know how to get answers to your questions if the handbook is not
available or insufficient; that you have answered all correspondence
from teacher and principal; that you have written a list of questions
that you want to ask the teacher; that you have noted your child's statement about his enjoyment of school, his participation in school activities, and the quality of his work. Bring written notes and leave them
with the teacher if necessary, so that he or she can review them later.

During the conference find out whether your child is at grade level
in all of the major subjects. Discuss whether recent achievement testing
has been done. Find out what areas need more work. Inspect samples of
your child's deskwork and find out what kinds of work he should be
bringing home. Ask about any changes in learning or classroom behavior. Finally, review the need for any additional special services and ask
the teacher how you can be of most help to him or her.

The first few minutes of conferences are crucial. Your actions and
the teacher's actions tend to reflect underlying attitudes. If the teacher
starts the conference with a list of the latest complaints about how your
child is ruining school for classmates, the teacher's attitude needs to be

dealt with immediately. In the same way, your warmth and friendliness toward the teacher must be made apparent in the first few moments of the conference to help set the tone for a cooperative relationship.

• TELEPHONE CALLS. Telephone contact is fast and convenient. It has the additional advantage of being direct, so that you and the teacher can communicate without interruption and in privacy. It is best if done after school hours by prearrangement, so that the teacher is more free to talk. If you call the school in the morning, it may be best to leave the message with the school secretary rather than to try conversing at length with the teacher. Use the phone to relay a quick warning to the teacher in the morning if your child is having a bad day, so that he or she can adjust expectations and activities for your child. After-school telephone calls can be used to provide a personal touch to your expressions of appreciation to the teacher whenever your child comes home particularly happy or encouraged about what occurred at school that day.

• NOTES. Brief written notes can flow between home and school. The teacher can send special instructions for the child, explanations of homework assignments, or descriptions of classroom events. You can use notes to inform the teacher about special family situations, about behavior changes that you have noticed in the child, or about other matters.

It is important not to overdo communicating with the teacher. A reasonably frequent flow of communication will probably help the teacher to understand your child. An excess of letters and phone calls, however, may cause harmful attitudes to develop; the teacher may start thinking of you as an overprotective parent more to be avoided than paid attention to.

Arranging Home/School Coordination

An important area of cooperation is the handling of homework. Provide a quiet place for study, encourage your child to set aside a specific time for doing homework, and give your help when needed to assist him with difficult parts of the assignment. Some simple arrangement can be developed for making sure that the child does the homework. A small notebook can be used exclusively for homework assignments, and the child should be expected to show it at home each evening. If no homework has been assigned, have the teacher indicate that fact in the notebook.

One variety of homework is spill-over from the work which was supposed to have been completed in the classroom during the school day. If your child brings home unfinished paperwork often, check into the situation. The teacher may not be checking thoroughly enough to see that your child completes the assigned work during regular class time. The assignments may be too long or too tedious, or they may be too difficult for your child. If so, arrange with the teacher that your child will complete all unfinished work at home, provided that difficulty level and lengths of assignments are appropriate. It is important to teach your child that he cannot avoid correctly geared school work by being slow at it.

In some cases the teacher may decide that homework would not be helpful. Be willing to support this decision if it appears sound. A hyperactive child does not *always* have to have homework, even if the child is behind his classmates in basic skills or knowledge.

Your child may benefit from a few minutes spent each night at home in a tutoring situation. Most teachers are delighted if parents aid the educational process by reviewing certain types of material with their children at home. After you have seen what the teacher's approach is and what he or she is trying to teach your child, try to arrange a way to review or reinforce the teaching effort at home. Coordinate your efforts with the teacher. Such a joint project brings you meaningfully into the educational process, makes you a more knowledgeable member of your child's resource team, helps you see your child's progress, helps you understand your child's difficulties, and helps your child see home and school as a cooperating and coordinated unit. Although not a suitable plan for all parents, this type of arrangement can also promote family closeness. Home study sessions should be short; from ten to thirty minutes is plenty for most families. Drill and practice can be made into fun activities, such as flash card games, if necessary.

Another important aspect of home/school cooperation pertains to the treatment of your child's hyperactivity. The teacher can arrange some sort of signal to remind your child about medication or nutrition management, without drawing unnecessary attention to him. The teacher's support for nutrition management can often be obtained by explaining the approach in terms of controlling your child's sensitivities by managing what he does and does not eat.

The Teacher's Role

Ideally the teacher will take a helpful attitude toward your child, which will be reflected in the approach the teacher uses toward other helpers.

Coordinating with Other Helpers

The physician in his office and the teacher in the classroom each probably make valid and accurate observations within their own settings. Each can, however, enlarge the point of view of the other. The physician needs to know about classroom behavior, and the teacher needs to know whether the child is receiving treatment through medication or nutrition management.

There is a danger of overlapping into each other's area of competence. Many teachers therefore are very careful never to diagnose that a child is hyperactive and never to recommend that the parents seek treatment for the hyperactivity. On the other hand, many physicians hesitate to communicate directly with the school without the specific consent of the parents.

You may have to position yourself between the physician and the school, serving as the communication link between the two helping resources. There is a danger of loss of confidentiality in written messages from the physician to the school. There is also a danger that messages from the physician will not filter down to the school personnel who really need them. One solution is to have the physician make written reports addressed "To Whom It May Concern" and hand them to you. It then becomes *your* responsibility to see that they get into the right hands, and *only* the right hands, at school. If more direct communication is needed, suggest a conference with the teacher and the physician both present.

Giving the child medication to take to school carries the risk of its loss, theft, or sale. A better method is to leave a supply of medication under appropriate adult supervision at school. The physician can help to negotiate this arrangement.

Most school personnel welcome any help in understanding the special needs of a hyperactive student. The mental health specialist can be involved in major decisions regarding your child's school progress.

In many cases it is wise to inform the concerned teacher that your child is participating in counseling or psychotherapy. If there are conflicts or difficulties in the classroom, the teacher can ask your child to discuss them at the next session with the mental health specialist. The teacher can also inform the mental health specialist of any changes in your child's behavior which indicate progress or regression.

The mental health specialist should be able to consult with the school faculty about hyperactivity or similar issues, providing new ideas during school conferences with the teacher and both parents present.

Accepting Your Child's Hyperactivity

The concerned teacher's attitude is one that conceives of your child as a precious human being, with all the lovability and all the needs that everyone has. Such a teacher will be a firm and kind person who understands hyperactivity and wants to learn more about it. He or she will display friendliness and warmth toward your child. The hyperactivity will be regarded as a challenge, an opportunity to expand teaching skills in order to reach a child with special needs. It takes little skill to teach a completely eager and capable student; teaching a hyperactive child takes considerable skill, however, and thus is a more fulfilling experience for the teacher who takes the profession seriously and who has a sense of mission.

When your child fails at a task, the teacher will be self-critical, questioning the teaching method and the academic demands that have been made. He or she will not jump to easy, superficial conclusions such as thinking that your child is lazy, uncooperative, or unteachable, but instead will ask questions like: "What could I be doing that would be slowing this student's progress? Was the material too demanding? Did the activity lack structure? Did the activity flood this child with too many choices to make? Was this child's perception fragmented, so that distractibility became too great?"

In general, the teacher will allow your child to express his uniqueness as long as it does not hinder academic or social progress or create disruption for others. The teacher will not be constantly trying to get your child to stifle himself, but instead, will be helping your child to find legitimate avenues for his self-expression.

Accommodating to Your Child's Hyperactivity

The academic program that your child's school offers depends on a number of factors. Your child might be placed in a regular classroom. Accommodations to your child's academic needs will consist of modifications in routine classroom procedures. The teacher will engineer most of them without outside help, but should ask for such help when it is needed and available.

A popular approach in elementary schools is the learning center, in which the child has a choice of several activities during the school day. Centers or areas of the classroom are devoted to various projects and activities. In some cases the learning center method of organizing the classroom works well with hyperactive children, and in some cases it does not. The child, the teacher, the classroom setting, and the organization of the centers are all important and variable factors.

Another academic approach is the special self-contained classroom, in which the physical structure and teaching methods are geared especially for learning-disabled and hyperactive children, or other children with special types of school difficulties. Usually the instructor has had special training in this area and has audio-visual and educational devices and equipment not ordinarily available in regular classrooms. Your child, however, may not want to be in such a class, for fear of being singled out, being given special assignments, or being labeled as different by the other children at school.

In general, hyperactive children need the extra help that is available in a special class, and they have difficulty functioning in a regular classroom without special accommodations to their learning disabilities. This conflict between academic goals and the hyperactive students' social and emotional needs is sometimes resolved by a compromise, the resource room.

The resource room is maintained by a person with special training and is made available to children with academic difficulties for a short period of time each day rather than being the children's only classroom. The children may come individually or in small groups to the resource room. In schools in which students frequently pass from room to room, hyperactive children can visit the resource room as a matter of course, and their visits will be relatively unnoticed by their schoolmates.

Whether your child is in a regular classroom, a special all-day classroom, or a resource room which can be visited for short periods, the school system probably has a consultant to the teachers who can assist in arranging subject matter and teaching methods to suit your child's abilities.

One characteristic of most school programs for hyperactive and learning-disabled children is the necessity of a high ratio of adults to students. If only one adult is available to teach the students, a high ratio is obtained by having only a few students in the class. If additional adults can serve as teacher aides, either on a paid or a volunteer basis, the number of children in the class can be increased. If several aides are available, it is best that *one* of them work exclusively with your child on a regular basis, rather than having several aids rotate the responsibility of assisting your child.

Any switch in schools can be difficult because of the flood of new situations and new people with which your child must deal. The transition is even more difficult when the style of class scheduling is different between the two schools. The child who transfers from a quiet, small elementary school (in which most of each day was spent with one teacher) to a junior high or middle school with hundreds of other students is put under severe stress. Besides the many new faces, there are dozens of new teachers, complicated class rotation schedules, many more rules, confusing lunchtime procedure, and a host of other pressures.

To aid in transition periods, and at other times, your child needs a personal relationship with a counselor, a guide teacher, a principal, or another adult in the school building. Your child needs to be able to talk to someone about his feelings, without fear of being lectured or of being dismissed as a nuisance. This caring adult can help your child focus on ways of improving school adjustment, including new approaches to solving school-related difficulties.

Learning More About Your Child

The effective teacher will want to obtain a brief history from you about your child's interests, favorite activities, special talents, and other personal bits of information. The teacher will particularly want to know about the types of situations which tend to trigger negative reactions in your child, so that he or she can avoid exposing your child to such conditions. What your child's other teachers have found to be effective in terms of disciplinary as well as instructional techniques will also be important.

The teacher will want to know how your child relates to the rest of his family. Particularly in relation to brothers and sisters who attend the same school, your child's place within the family structure will be an important piece of information for the teacher, who may want to interview your child for the purpose of obtaining a full picture of how your child sees the family and the world at large.

Despite his loud voice and talkativeness, your child may not have developed the ability to express and communicate his feelings clearly to others. Through the medium of self-expressive art forms, the teacher can gain insight into your child's current emotional state that he may not otherwise be able to express in a clear or useful way. If your child seems to be angry one day, for example, the teacher may offer some paint or other art medium with an instruction such as: "Paint a picture of what you are mad about" or "Draw a picture that shows someone who feels the way you do today."

The teacher will want to learn your child's particular styles of dealing with potentially threatening or stressful tasks, so that he or she can find ways to stimulate your child's wholehearted participation in the class. The teacher will be interested in what you have noticed about your child's avoidance techniques as well as what you have heard about them from previous teachers.

If your child has developed a fear of failure, gives up quickly, or refuses to try tasks that look challenging, he has probably also developed some other tell-tale signs that indicate he is afraid to take risks. This pattern of behavior is the fourth goal or purpose of misbehavior, as discussed in Chapter 12. Particularly in a situation in which the quality of his work will be judged, your child may be tempted to give up or may not try to do the work. Common comments among hyperactive children who display this type of misbehavior are these: "I can't do this now," "I already know how to do this," "I haven't been able to do it before, so why try now?" "I'll do it at home . . . tomorrow . . . later . . . in a little bit . . . as soon as I finish this other thing," and "I did it last

year, so why do I have to do it again this year?" The teacher will be
alert for such indications of discouragement.

Your child may try to avoid academic stress by finding excuses to
leave the classroom. Getting drinks from a water fountain, going to the
bathroom, wandering the halls, going to the library, going to the locker,
visiting a counselor, and hunting for items like bandages and facial tissue are common excuses. Some popular excuses for avoiding work
while still inside the classroom are breaking pencils, combing hair, and
looking for papers. The teacher will note any such actions by your
child.

Perhaps sending a note home each day with a summary of homework
assignments, having a routine progress report sent back and forth between home and school, or some other system has been useful in the
past. Any such special techniques that have been tried by other teachers will also be of interest to your child's current teacher.

Chapter 11

Effective Teaching Approaches

Your child's teachers exert a profound influence in the classroom which, in many instances, you can neither modify nor prevent. For as many as six hours a day they supervise and direct a number of transactions which cause varying degrees of stress in your child.

The teacher's influence on your child can be said to be of three kinds: personal encouragement, social skills, and academic training.

Providing Encouragement

With the right words and actions, the teacher can raise the sagging self-esteem that could cripple your child educationally and emotionally.

Guarding Your Child's Self-Esteem

The successful teacher knows that every child needs to feel successful and will, therefore, create opportunities for your child to achieve a sense of satisfaction and accomplishment. Immediate acknowledgment of effort may be indicated by the placing of colorful hand-drawn smiles, stars, or stickers on your child's papers. The teacher may send a personal letter of encouragement to your child. Such a letter would be treasured and would serve as an excellent way for the teacher to help maintain your child's interest and involvement in class activities. The teacher's method of verbally acknowledging your child's effort should ideally be similar to the types of encouraging methods described in Chapter 5.

Touch is very important in giving any child the sense of being nurtured, cared for, and worthwhile. The teacher should try to greet your child each day and find unobtrusive ways to touch him briefly, perhaps with a light pat on the shoulder.

The effective teacher knows that the best ways to teach responsibility are to expect it and to create situations in which it can be displayed. He or she will assign responsibilities with the expectation that your child will be able to carry them out or will at least try hard to do so. Even if the child is not completely successful, the teacher should respond in a supportive and encouraging way.

The teacher should not display the classroom work of only a handful of favored students. Instead, *all* students' work should be displayed around the room, including your child's work.

The teacher should be careful to avoid situations which would embarrass or belittle your child, including labeling him as hyperactive and mentioning his treatment program.

Using Your Child's Strengths

The successful teacher should capitalize on your child's strengths and use them as the foundation for his classroom participation. The most successful teaching approaches maximize these strengths to help compensate for weaknesses while simultaneously attempting to strengthen the weak areas. The multi-modal approach discussed later in this chapter is excellent for accomplishing both objectives. The modes in which your child already functions well should be used for accomplishing the learning, while the weaker modes should be strengthened by being paired with the stronger modes. The teacher should channel learning to the strong modes when your child needs an uplifting and easy assignment; the weaker modes should be used when the child appears to have the necessary confidence to risk having some difficulties and errors.

If your child likes to draw, the teacher should allow a time for drawing at the end of those class periods in which he was particularly well behaved or completed his work satisfactorily. The teacher should urge your child to share his strengths and talents with the group. If your child has special knowledge about a certain topic, the wise teacher might ask him to work with another student in making a class presentation on that topic.

The teacher should give your child opportunities to follow and pursue his interests and to express them in constructive ways. Assigned work should be within your child's capacity so that he can experience the satisfaction of accomplishment.

Under these circumstances, your child's talents will be utilized to their best advantage, both in terms of academic advancement and improved social relationships.

Pacing Your Child's Work

The productive teacher will take one step at a time, dividing the assigned work into units, such as three ten-minute assignments rather than one thirty-minute assignment. That way, your child will be able to complete each unit before moving ahead to the next one. Each succeeding unit should involve a slightly more difficult or advanced stage of learning, so that the learning process can be graduated.

This procedure makes each task seem achievable and allows your child to concentrate fully on each one before taking on the next. He will be able to organize his thinking and concentration for each step without being distracted and overwhelmed by concerns about the total cluster of new concepts involved in the complete lesson. The task therefore will seem less difficult, less confusing, and less frightening to your child than if it had been presented as one large assignment. The trait of distractibility automatically dictates that each particular unit of learning should be small, calling for only a little expenditure of time and effort.

The creative teacher will avoid overloading your child, introducing a few concepts at a time. After each new group of concepts is introduced, it should be reviewed, so that the child can be tested to see if he has really acquired, absorbed, and retained the new knowledge. A few more concepts can then be introduced. The next review may be cumulative, including previously learned material as well as the most recently introduced. New knowledge is thus presented, reviewed, absorbed, tested, and integrated with previously learned material in a step-by-step fashion.

The teacher should allow your child to complete one type of activity before starting another. For example, your child might be asked to first copy *all* of the arithmetic problems, then work on them. Similarly, your child may be asked to copy subtraction problems first, then solve them, then copy and solve all addition problems, and so forth.

The course of progress should be from simple tasks to complex ones, from mastery to challenge.

The teacher should not try to force your child to read more, write faster, or copy arithmetic problems more quickly if the slowness is a result of learning disabilities. Your child will be responsible for all as-

signed work, but the watchful teacher should see that the amount of it
does not overwhelm him. If your child is slow at writing, for example,
the total amount of assignments demanding writing skill should be
lowered, but the child's grade should not be. To avoid unfairly penal-
izing your child, the teacher should make appropriate accommodations
on tests. They can be given orally or by tape recorder if your child's
lack of reading and writing skills would be an unfair burden. As long as
your child is devoting earnest effort, the teacher should feel free to decrease the workload and grade on effort, not quantity.

Using Grading Systems Carefully

Grading is an important consideration, because grades can be an extremely discouraging, destructive process which hinders rather than
helps children's academic progress. If your child has academic problems, grades can be a special threat.

It is not a good idea for either the parent or the teacher to put a lot of
emphasis on grades. The successful teacher will not emphasize them
and will not use them to shame your child into increasing his classroom
participation. The teacher will know that the most important factors
are your child's enjoyment of the work and the amount of effort that he
puts into the work. These are the effective criteria of your child's academic success and they should be recognized and supported by the
teacher and by you.

Grades must be considered in relation to their function. If their purpose is to inform parents of the child's academic progress, then they
must reflect the quantity and quality of the child's work in the
classrooom. If their purpose is to help motivate the child, they should
emphasize his effort, cooperativeness, and successes.

The teacher should grade on concept knowledge rather than on aspects of the work which are irrelevant. For example, there should be no
grading penalty for miscopied arithmetic problems if your child has a
perceptual difficulty. There should be no grade for neatness of the
work if lack of neatness results simply from poor coordination.

Sometimes the teacher is not free to make such independent decisions about the use of the school's grading system. Urge the teacher to
get blanket approval for special handling of grading your child if such
permission is needed.

The teacher should accompany the grades with an indication of the successful and positive aspects of your child's classroom production. When writing the grade on your child's paper, for example, the thoughtful teacher will circle all of the *correct* answers. An encouraging comment should accompany the grade, regardless of how high or low it is.

Helping Your Child Socially

Training in social skills is just as important as training in academic subjects. Many of the difficulties your child may experience at school involve relationships with other children and with school personnel. The observant teacher will use opportunities that occur each day for teaching social skills to your child and to your child's classmates.

Helping Your Child Be a Part of the Group

The teacher should develop a group spirit and a sense of cohesiveness in the class. Competition and favoritism will be eliminated, to be replaced by cooperativeness among the students. Classmates will support each other and the teacher will aid the children in coming to a classwide consensus on issues. The class should hold regular meetings to make various decisions. At these meetings every student should feel free to express concerns, discuss issues, and outline needs with regard to the teacher, other students, or the school. There should be free and open communication and trust between teacher and students, generating a spirit of mutual cooperation for the common good.

The class discussions should include concerns involving the students' relations with each other. The teacher, in turn, should use these discussions to train the children in how to relate to each other in supportive and positive ways.

When intervention is necessary in a difficult moment, the wise teacher will not label an action by your child in a condemnatory way. By privately explaining your child's hyperactivity to individual classmates who are temporarily frustrated or angry, the teacher can help your child to be accepted by the class. A statement such as, "It is sometimes hard for Billy to sit still and to avoid talking to you," can make your child's relations with his classmates smoother.

Preventing Misbehavior

The teacher who is successful with your child will place a great deal of emphasis on preventing misbehavior and will use the classroom's structure and procedures for that purpose. Such a teacher will know that effective classroom discipline must rest on a positive, happy atmosphere and a spirit of caring and cooperation between teacher and students.

The seats should be movable so that their positions can be changed quickly. The positions of the students with respect to each other can therefore be rapidly rearranged whenever a disruption threatens to take place.

The teacher should have spare pencils, paper, and facial tissues handy for minor upsets in routine.

There should be a neutral time-out area to which your child can go at those moments when he needs to calm down. The area might have some games, art supplies, or other materials to help him overcome pent-up feelings and to occupy him whenever he is unable to participate in the regular classroom activity.

There should be provisions for music that the teacher can turn on and off as a behavior control measure. Various other aspects of ordinary classroom procedures can also serve to prevent misbehavior. The teacher may use the lights as a behavior control measure, primarily as a signal for a change in activity.

The effective teacher will know that routine is important to your child and will write a schedule on the blackboard, for example, outlining each day's activities.

The thinking teacher will not overwhelm your child with the responsibility of making too many choices in a short period of time. Instead, he or she will allow your child to make choices gradually, starting with a simple choice between only two options.

The teacher should know that your child must always be permitted to finish speaking when he has started to say something, even if the teacher would like him to stop. Recognizing that this rigidity is not a defiance of authority but is, instead, a symptom of your child's hyperactivity, the teacher will wait politely until your child has finished talking, so that he will not experience needless frustration in being interrupted.

Using Humane Disciplinary Methods

Misbehavior by students is an expected part of any classroom situation. The wise teacher will deal with it immediately and not resent its disruption of classroom routine. He or she will try to resolve potential conflict situations in a supportive, helpful, and instructive fashion.

The teacher will recognize which of the four mistaken goals of misbehavior (described in Chapter 12) your child is displaying and will counter the misbehavior accordingly. The teacher will realize that a negative situation need not be handled negatively. He or she will help your child discriminate between acceptable and unacceptable behavior in the classroom without rejecting, criticizing, or blaming him but by firmly refusing to accept his misbehavior as legitimate. This confrontation with your child should be done in a positive way. A signal such as clearing the throat twice or tapping a pencil might be prearranged as a reminder to your child to return his full attention to the assigned classwork. Other gentle and unobtrusive reminder signals might also be agreed upon in advance, with direct input from the child, to curb his temptations to misbehave.

Effective solutions create lasting harmony for the future rather than merely providing stop-gap day-to-day truces. The effective teacher knows that your child can best learn how to arrive at these solutions through honest and direct feedback from the other children. The class will be instructed in confrontation methods because the teacher will want your child to learn the necessary social realities. Left to their own devices, your child's classmates may use only destructive forms of confrontation: physical attack, getting revenge, rejecting your child, criticizing, name-calling, and so forth. The teacher will teach the other students how to confront each other (including your child) in a constructive way that will lead to settlement rather than prolonging of the conflict (see Chapter 8).

Though time is in short supply for even the most successful and effective teachers, it can be wisely invested by your child's teacher in the use of the disciplinary techniques described in Chapters 12 and 13. Stop-gap measures save time for the moment, but in the long run they cause more problems than they solve.

In grades beyond the primary level, the teacher might occasionally involve the entire class in disciplinary situations. If your child misbehaves for the purpose of getting undue attention from his classmates, for example, the teacher may instruct the class to be unimpressed by his antics, so that the goal of his misbehavior will not be achieved.

For your child, the opportunity to move around and be physically active during the lunch period is usually very important. Accordingly, if extra work in the classroom is needed, the teacher will not deprive your child of recess. Instead, he will be asked to remain after school, to come in early the next day, or to do the work during another class period.

Your child will also welcome the chance to use time-out areas. The time-out area can be in the classroom, but it may also be elsewhere in the school. If your child tends to build up a significant amount of anger or restlessness in the classroom, the opportunity to go to a gymnasium and to bounce on tumbling mats can help a great deal in preventing misbehavior. Such an arrangement, of course, must have the approval of all involved school personnel. Forcing your child to stifle and hide these needs may simply result in his trying to use them for socially destructive purposes, such as creating disciplinary problems in the classroom.

The school is rejecting its obligation to educate your child if it suspends him without first having exhausted all other approaches. Research has found suspension to be especially damaging to hyperactive children. It isolates them and puts them into a destructive and repetitive cycle of frustration, failure, misbehavior, and retaliation from others. It is a one-way, dead-end street. Suspending your child from school is therefore *not* one of the disciplinary methods preferred by an effective teacher.

Educating Your Child in Social Skills

Many parents of hyperactive children have selected schools in which the classrooms are quiet and orderly, only to discover that too much academic pressure was put on their children and social and emotional growth was neglected or weakened. There may have been a lack of interaction among students or a lack of attention given by the teacher to social and emotional factors.

The classroom of the successful teacher of a hyperactive child is quiet and orderly, and there will be no heavy academic pressure. Academic requirements must be balanced with information on how to get along with oneself and others. In addition to presenting educational material, the teacher will assist your child in developing social skills. The teacher will try to involve your child in a social awareness program, small group discussions, self-concept exploration, or similar experiences. Some of these programs include pamphlets, tape recordings, and other devices to educate students in basic principles of interpersonal relationships, conflict solving, and self-esteem.

In addition to direct instruction in these matters, the creative teacher will also be a role model who demonstrates effective social skills. Class meetings are important in this regard.

Using Effective Educational Methods

Many instructional techniques have recently been developed for use with hyperactive and learning-disabled children. Almost every aspect of teaching style, classroom arrangement, and educational material can be directed toward benefiting the hyperactive child in the classroom.

Using Special Instruction Techniques

The best type of education for your child accommodates to his strengths and weaknesses at the beginning of his school experience and continues to do so throughout his academic career. Most hyperactive children, however, do not receive such special instruction until their learning handicaps have started to become apparent. Sometimes the school personnel do not display sufficient concern. They may fail to realize that relying solely on ordinary classroom methods of instruction will not work. The typical hyperactive child can be several years behind classmates in various academic skills, often necessitating remedial methods.

Because of his frequently slow progress in writing and reading, as well as his impaired ability to organize thoughts into effective priorities, note-taking is usually a difficult task for the hyperactive child. The lecture method of instruction thus unfairly penalizes him. Your child may need to receive instruction in a format other than a lecture. Instead of broadcasting homework assignments to the entire class, the teacher may have to give your child individual instruction. The same principle may also apply to desk work done in the classroom.

An especially effective technique involves using more than one of your child's senses in the learning experience. Combinations of sight, hearing, touch, movement (kinesthesis), taste, and smell can be involved simultaneously to create an integrated experience. This use of several senses at the same time permits learning to take place faster and more effectively than by using just one sense at a time. For certain limited learning situations, this approach is the preferred method.

This process, called multi-modal learning, can be illustrated in teaching a first-grade child the sound of the letter M. A typical multi-modal approach would be to have the child say "mmm" after hearing the teacher say it, as the child traces with his fingertip on a large piece of sandpaper a large letter M which is painted on the sandpaper. The child *hears* the teacher and himself say the sound of the letter, *moves* his hand, arm, and mouth, *sees* the large letter on the sandpaper and *feels* the sandpaper with his fingertip. Even though your child may have poor coordination, a multi-modal approach involving movement will be helpful. Multi-modal learning is the ideal, but it may not be practical in some classrooms because of other demands made on the teacher.

By writing the assignment on the blackboard for the children to copy, the successful teacher can reinforce verbal instructions. Parents can also use the blackboard at home. Using a typewriter at home or at school can involve your child in a helpful multi-modal experience, especially if he repeats aloud what he is typing.

One-to-one teaching is often very effective with a hyperactive child, but unfortunately it usually has to be severely rationed in most school systems. The principle is nevertheless valid, and a successful teacher will try to arrange some method of one-to-one teaching for your child. Your child will make more progress if he has five minutes of individual attention and help, and then spends the remaining twenty-five minutes working by himself, than if he had to work as part of the class group (lecture method) for thirty minutes. The process of providing one-to-one instruction for your child will be much easier if aides are available to the teacher.

Providing individualized instruction does not always mean forcing your child to work alone. Assignments can be given so that your child's work is part of a coordinated class activity, but is given to your child only.

The hyperactive trait of seeming to know something one minute but forgetting it a few minutes later can move a teacher to doubt how much your child has actually learned. The teacher should make practice and drill interesting for your child, so that distractibility doesn't destroy the effect of the exercises. The effective teacher will distinguish between memorizing and understanding. Drilling encourages memorizing and should be given as the *last* step in any newly learned material, only *after* your child has demonstrated his understanding of the new material.

Adjusting Your Child's Curriculum

The curriculum should be individualized, so that your child can be provided with the most important courses and topics. In order to create your child's curriculum, the teacher will want to measure abilities such as reading, cursive writing, spelling, mathematics, and other relevant areas. Ideally the teacher will also want to hear your ideas about curriculum adjustment.

The effective teacher will try to teach at approximately your child's level of achievement. Curriculum planning should provide experiences by which your child can exercise his abilities without becoming frustrated. An extremely easy school assignment may not be challenging or, in the long run, even satisfying. Tasks that are too challenging are also not satisfying and may quickly lead your child to stop trying. In this way your child's self-confidence can be developed and he can experience the joy of accomplishment and the momentum of success. The effective teacher will try to dilute challenging material with enough easily done work so that the total experience is not too stressful for your child.

Neither too much nor too little help will be offered by the truly effective teacher. The need to repeat such admonitions as "figure it out" or "try harder" may indicate that your child has already reached his frustration level because of the difficulty of the work. At such moments, one-to-one attention and instruction should be given. Help from the teacher should be available to your child, but withheld until he makes an earnest attempt to learn through his own efforts.

One part of your child's curriculum that merits special attention is physical education. For early adolescent hyperactive children, gym class is often one of the most troublesome and embarrassing times of the school day. Disrobing, wearing uniforms, displaying physical coordination, and other activities of physical education classes can be very difficult challenges. Your child needs opportunities to release energy and a physical education class is such an opportunity, but many physical education courses fall short of their potential by not offering much more than competitive team sports.

Some of the results of your child's participation in a truly effective and creative physical education program will be release of energy, control of breathing, improvement of coordination and muscle, sharpened sense of balance, and knowledge of exercise and nutrition principles. These results can occur if the physical education curriculum includes such activities as dance, relaxation training, structured exercise programs, posture and body movement training, and individual sports such as swimming, bowling, tennis, skating, golfing, racquetball, handball, and archery.

Accommodating to Your Child's Distractibility

The effective teacher will aim for a small class size or a high adult-to-student ratio in a more crowded classroom. He or she will know that anything that is out of place can be distracting to your child and can preoccupy him. Ideally, there should be a special section set aside for the hyperactive child, where classroom supplies, particularly those used by your child, would always be in the same place; the blackboard should be cleaned at the start of each day; there should be no mobiles dangling from the ceiling and no clusters of brightly colored pictures on the wall.

The teacher should act calm and unhurried, avoiding quick or extreme movements of the hands, fingers, or pencils. Pointers should be moved slowly and smoothly, rather than in rapid starting and stopping motions.

Your child's desk should be in an area that is relatively free from distractions and where supervision is easy, so that he can be given instructions quickly. Depending on the physical arrangement of the classroom, his desk might be next to the desks of quiet children, next to the teacher's desk, or in a corner, separated by some sort of partition to narrow your child's range of immediate vision. It might face a wall rather than the classroom. It should be away from windows, doors, and the room's high traffic areas.

If the desk is in a corner, a bookcase, a blanket draped over a rope, sides of a large shipping carton or specially constructed opaque screens might be used to isolate it. It might become your child's "office" where he can work peacefully. Under no circumstances should this special seating arrangement be used as a punishment for your child, although sometimes other children might use it as a time-out area. Your child may have to be taught the need for this type of arrangement, that it is intended to allow him to concentrate more fully on classwork, and that his enjoyment and participation in the class will be enhanced. The teacher should explain these concepts to the other children without embarrassing or labeling your child.

Although a desk that is screened somewhat from the others in the classroom may seem at first to hinder any child's sense of belonging, the opposite effect usually occurs if the arrangement is handled properly by the teacher. This special plan allows a much higher level of academic success and therefore enthusiasm for school than would occur if it were not made for your child. His academic success paves the way for his social success, and his behavior is better controlled and more tolerable to classmates when the seating arrangements control distractibility in this fashion.

Sometimes your child may be so distracted by the background and format of a page in a book that the ability to concentrate on the word or idea being taught is lost. The teacher should help by isolating the item from its background and writing the word or phrase on the blackboard or on a separate piece of paper. Non-essential material should be covered, and your child should be encouraged to use a pointer, marker, or hand-held cardboard border. Reading machines might also be used.

Your child's desk should be clear and uncluttered. The only items on it should be those necessary to complete each assignment as it is given. At other times, the desk should be cleared of all objects, with the possible exception of a brightly colored contrast mat, which can help limit his visual field during desk work.

Accommodating to Your Child's Constant Movement

Your child may become fidgety when asked to remain still and to focus his attention over an extended period of time. A switch to vigorous activity may be needed in order for him to discharge his need for constant movement. The successful teacher will know that any sustained sitting, even in circumstances which are enjoyable for other children, may cause a build-up of restlessness. Active movement will be necessary before your child will be ready to concentrate fully on academic work. The teacher will find opportunities for movement, rather than trying to force him to stifle that need.

Attempts should be made to schedule some active periods in the routine daily classroom activities. Some special arrangement should be made for your child, so that leaving the desk will not always be an infraction of the rules. He may be permitted, for example, to do desk work one page at a time, turning each page in to the teacher before receiving the next page. Rest periods can be active periods for your child, especially if they follow quiet times involving a high amount of concentration. Music may have a calming effect on your child, and might be used by the teacher during the transition from an active period to one of quiet concentration.

The teacher should also try to arrange for vigorous activity for your child during the lunch period. If legitimate vigorous physical activity cannot be built into the daily routine, the teacher should try to excuse your child from the classroom for those brief periods when his restlessness has built up. He also might be allowed to assist cafeteria, custodial, or office staff for short periods during the day in order to channel his need for activity in a constructive direction.

SECTION FIVE

GUIDING YOUR CHILD

In their search for disciplinary techniques that work, parents of hyperactive children often go from one extreme to the other, from being very harsh to being very flexible at different times. The result is that the parents develop several bad habits and gradually surrender the leadership of their hyperactive child. The behavior of the child, meanwhile, grows steadily worse. Bedtimes, meal times, shopping trips, times when company is present, and times when the parent is on the telephone become occasions for marked misbehavior by the child.

The first chapter in this section discusses the bad habits that can occur in disciplinary strategy and how to prevent their development. It also describes an approach to child discipline that allows the parents to remain strong and continue their leadership position. The second chapter describes many tools of parental discipline, so that they have more techniques and more options to choose from in dealing with their child's misbehavior. The third chapter discusses how to structure and supervise the child's play activities and how to select toys that will help him learn to play contentedly and peaceably.

The first two chapters are applicable to children of any age level, with or without behavior problems.

Chapter 12

Laying the Groundwork for Discipline

Hyperactive children misbehave a great deal. Their misbehavior, like that of any other children, can be understood and it can be dealt with by effective disciplinary methods. Your hyperactive child has the same social purposes for his misbehavior as does the misbehaving child who is not hyperactive.

Your efforts to prevent misbehavior and to lay the groundwork for effective discipline must be constant. Do not wait until a treatment program has been fully established. Your leadership of your child is a responsibility that should precede as well as follow any attempt to treat him by medication or nutrition management.

Use Your Leadership to Prevent Misbehavior

Often your child may seem to deserve negative reactions to his misbehavior when, however, his greatest need is for more love. When most messages your child receives are negative, discipline is likely to be ineffective. When any child knows that many of the times his parents talk to him he will be yelled at, bossed, or criticized, he has little reason to want to please them.

Develop a process by which your child can negotiate with all of the other family members for what he wants. Knowing that he will be heard and that his needs will be paid attention to assures him of his acceptance within the family. Regular family meetings for this purpose can help; guidelines for them were given in Chapter 9.

Try to keep the child's stimulation level low by having him play with only one friend at a time, rather than with a large group of children. Be willing, however, to allow a larger play group as your child shows increased ability to play easily with more children. Don't expose him needlessly to large groups in other situations. Take extra precautions about taking your child to supermarkets, parties, long trips, and stores with delicate items on the shelves. Leaving him without supervision when you are entertaining visitors in your home may also be inviting trouble.

Try to keep your child occupied with one thing at a time, rather than giving him multiple stimulation. You may want to give your child one toy at a time from a closed toy box, for example. When he is working at a table, clear it of all objects except the one with which he is working. Turn off a television or radio that is creating needless background noise.

Designate a room or part of a room as your child's special place where he can do art work, work in crafts, play with toys, and busy himself safely and without overstimulation.

Some hyperactive children are bothered by their sense of a lack of predictability in their responses and actions. Constancy becomes important to them, and they are reassured when the events at home are scheduled and predictable. Post schedules and routines for household activities, including a wall chart that lists chores for all family members. Try to give your home structure, quiet, and routine. If your home is orderly, with things in their proper places, your child will be less likely to become overstimulated or confused. Make changes slowly and gradually whenever possible. Deviations in routines or furniture arrangements should be announced ahead of time.

Time your requests to conform with your child's daily schedule, taking into account any flux in his moods. When you schedule an activity, consider your child's readiness for different types of experience at different times of day. If he is calmer in the morning than in the afternoon, for example, take him shopping with you during the morning.

When routines and scheduled activities are changed without advance warning, your child might need some special help. Explain the situation rather than leaving him surprised and confused, and avoid sudden terminations of his activities. Tell your child ahead of time whenever he must stop one activity in order to switch to a different one. It is better to say "five more turns" in order to bring a game to a close than to announce suddenly that the game is over.

Time your requests to come between rather than during your child's favorite television programs. Attach a time limit to your requests, so that your child has enough time to complete the current activity before being expected to start the new one.

Simple chores can be completed in short periods of time and a small timer may help give the child a sense of the passage of a few minutes. An instruction such as "You have ten minutes to pick up the toys," or "You have five minutes to complete your math problem," can be reinforced with the timer.

Provide supervision by being physically near the child. Touch him rather than giving only verbal direction from a distance. Avoid showering him with commands from the kitchen. Help structure the situation by directing and beginning his movement toward the desired activity. If you want toys to be picked up, for example, stand next to your child, pick up one toy, put it into the toy container, pick up another toy, hand it to him and say: "You pick up the rest of the toys now; I'll be back in five minutes to make sure they're all put away."

Make your requests clear by making a definite statement rather than asking a question. Avoid an apologetic "O.K.?" at the end of your statement. Don't haggle or negotiate about petty issues like an extra television program or trying a new food at the table. Take a firm position, state clearly and concisely what you want from your child, and stick by it.

Word your requests in a positive manner by stating what you want him to do, rather than what you want him not to do. In a theater, say "Whisper," rather than "Shhh, don't talk so loud." Say "Please carry your coat," rather than "Don't drag your coat."

Your child may have trouble understanding more than one request at a time. Make sure that you have his full attention, then state your request in simple, clear, one-concept statements. Have him repeat the request back to you if necessary. Speaking slowly is also helpful, as is writing out the request. Smaller children can be helped by little pictures on the list to help them understand any words they may not yet be able to read.

Sometimes your child may need a demonstration of new or difficult activities that he is being asked to engage in. Be willing to show him what to do, in addition to telling him.

Reminders may occasionally be needed. These reminders should not be scoldings. They should be a few simple words, given in a friendly tone of voice. Their purpose is to help keep your child's attention on his task while still leaving the final initiative up to him. You may want to suggest the next specific act in a sequence, such as: "Where is your towel?" or "What do you need to do next?" It is important not to overdo reminding him. He may quickly catch on to his opportunity to play helpless and get extra attention from you in the form of your constant reminding.

Discard Ineffective Methods

The ultimate goal of discipline is to train the child in self-control, not for him to be controlled by parents. In attempting to reach this goal, most parents mistakenly use one or more of these five ineffective methods of discipline: witchhunts, ignoring, piggyback messages, parent tantrums, and excessive punishment.

Witchhunts

Barging angrily into a situation to find the child who is to blame for the trouble is the first step in a witchhunt. A related error is assuming that your hyperactive child is completely responsible for the entire situation. Such mistakes increase family tension and decrease the amount of love that he feels. When you become so furious that you set out deliberately to "get" your child, then you are going on a witchhunt.

Instead, remove yourself temporarily from the stressful situation, size up the event, and move slowly back into the scene. Get explanations of the situation from the persons involved. Avoid raising your voice. Promise yourself that you will not try to pin the blame on anybody but that you will try instead to find a solution that is in line with the needs of everyone involved.

Ignoring

Ignoring is used too often and too early in a variety of disciplinary situations by many parents and teachers. In addition, a great many mental health professionals, who ought to know better, are unaware of the inefficiency of ignoring; they continue to recommend it as a cure-all, which it certainly is not.

Ignoring deprives the child of awareness of his true social impact on others. You may be frustrated by your child's actions, for example, but if you ignore them, you will not be communicating that fact to him and he will have missed a valuable lesson about the social consequences of his misbehavior. The isolation of the child that supposedly makes ignoring work as a disciplinary technique can backfire and deprive both parent and child of the processes that are crucial in helping him correct his misbehavior. Ignoring breaks off communication and decreases the ability to supervise and monitor the child's behavior. Ignoring implies rejection of the child and provides no chance to develop his self-esteem.

In order to understand why your child misbehaves, you must observe his actions and interpret the immediate results of the misbehavior in the context of the entire situation. Ignoring inhibits these processes and deprives you of the opportunity to recognize your child's hidden purposes for misbehaving.

Ignoring is very close to neglect and sometimes a child who is being ignored by a parent as a disciplinary measure will enter into an unsafe or life-threatening situation. At such a time, the parent is left feeling inadequate and foolish for not having better supervised the child. Under the pretense of ignoring, some parents continue to deny that their child is hyperactive.

Ignoring operates destructively on the continuing social process by creating too much ambiguity, confusing the situation with many possible misinterpretations. When you react to your child's misbehavior only by ignoring it, your child remains unclear about your attitude and emotional responses. Without clarification from you, he will probably assume the worst: that you no longer love him, that you have given up trying to set limits on his misbehavior, that you just don't care about him at all, or that he is too unimportant to care about.

Ignoring can allow problem behavior to continue without limits, creating an angry, frustrated parent who continually blames only the child for the stress in a situation. The stress would have been reduced, however, if the parent had confronted the child at the beginning rather than simply ignoring his continued misbehavior.

For the child who pushes and tests limits constantly, to ignore him is to invite him to *force* you to stop. Ignoring commonly results in an increase, rather than a decrease in a hyperactive child's misbehavior, particularly when the child's purpose is to display power or to get revenge (goals II and III, as discussed later in this chapter).

To avoid these pitfalls, use ignoring as a disciplinary technique only *after* you have explained your attitude about the misbehavior and have set your limits. Ignoring then becomes a demonstration of your intention to curtail your own further involvement in the misbehavior. Particularly when the child's goal is to gain attention (goal I, as discussed later in this chapter), he will learn that you will no longer be manipulated and that the situation is ended. The child who makes silly, irrelevant comments during a group discussion, for example, can be told that the discussion will proceed without recognition of any more of his remarks. The child will soon stop his attention-getting comments when they lose their usefulness and power through being ignored by the others in the discussion.

It is important to state your feelings about the misbehavior *only once*. If you state them again and again during each repeated attempt at misbehavior, you will be nagging rather than ignoring.

Ignoring must not be confused with your withdrawal from the scene, which can be a powerful and effective disciplinary technique. The use of withdrawal as a disciplinary technique is discussed in Chapter 13.

Piggyback Messages

Ten minutes before dinner, Mother called outside to Jimmy to come in and wash his hands for dinner; Jimmy promised to come home in a minute. Five minutes before dinner, Mother called again; again Jimmy promised to come in right away. As the food was being placed on the table, Mother called to Jimmy a third time; he assured her that he had heard and promised to be right in. Two minutes later, an angry parent yelled at a dawdling child and by threatening to deprive him of dinner was able to get him finally to come in to eat.

A piggyback message is one that is repeated, so that the child receives a series of similar or identical messages. If these messages are given all at once, as part of a single speech by the parent, it is called preaching. If a time delay occurs between each repeated message, as in the example above, it is called nagging. Most children start to receive piggyback messages when they are toddlers, in the form of constant "No" from parents.

Parents often have too much faith in words as tools for teaching and directing their children. But the more piggyback messages a child receives, the less powerful each message becomes. You will dilute the instructional and leadership effects of your words if you use too many identical piggyback messages.

Giving piggyback messages is one of the most common inefficient disciplinary efforts among parents of hyperactive children. The habit is easy to adopt, in part because of the child's weak memory for verbal instructions.

If any of these five circumstances occurs in your family, you are giving too many piggyback messages:

1. Does the hyperactive child nag, badger, and pester parents even though he knows that they won't back down on what they have already said?
2. Does the child wait for a reminder before taking action?
3. Does the child complain that parents are always asking him to do something, bothering him, and expressing dissatisfaction with his efforts?
4. Does the child become angry rather than grateful about reminders?
5. Do parents feel forced to give repeated messages because the child takes no action if no reminders are given?

To stop this inefficient method, begin communicating not only with words. Say what you have to say, but say it:

once
briefly
clearly
completely
firmly
calmly.

Follow through with a logical consequence or restructuring technique, as described in Chapter 13. Your disciplinary action should illustrate your intention or policy. Act; don't yak. If you absolutely must repeat a request, don't use the same words. In a calm voice say something like: "You already know what you have to do."

Parent Tantrums

This inefficient method occurs when you are at the end of your rope, as discussed in Chapter 6. Apologizing after having a tantrum over your child is better than leaving the scene without defusing the tense, emotional atmosphere. Obviously, not having the tantrum in the first place is best of all.

Parent tantrums are symptoms of being overwhelmed and out of control of the situation. They impede your child's learning about how to gain self-control, and teach him to have a tantrum of his own whenever others don't do what he wants them to do. Often the children who have learned to bully others into submission by having tantrums reflect the way they are treated by their parents.

If you have too few disciplinary tools, you are more likely to feel helpless in dealing with your child's misbehavior. Obtain more efficient disciplinary techniques, so that your confidence as a leader in your family will increase.

Excessive Punishment

When misbehavior occurs, many parents think they must do something to their child immediately in order to correct the situation and prevent further misbehavior. Punishment is usually a parent's first choice of action.

Often, however, you are not limited to doing something *to* your child; you can do things *with* or *for* him. Your response to the misbehavior can be directed at objects in the room, yourself, other people in the situation, or in other directions besides the child.

Disciplinary techniques are sometimes more effective if there is a delay rather than an immediate response to the misbehavior; your immediate response may tend to be impulsive, angry, and poorly thought out.

It is unrealistic to assume that any disciplinary technique will solve the problem and guarantee no further misbehavior. There is often no final solution to problems requiring discipline; therefore, the belief that you need to do something to your child immediately to dispose of the problem is more folly than fact.

A common myth is that punishment will teach children proper behavior and is the best answer to misbehavior. The truth is that many parents of a hyperactive child find to their amazement that the ordinary punishments, such as spanking, are pitifully ineffective in bringing about improvements in their child's behavior.

Parents use punishments for four major reasons: to maintain a sense of power and control over their children; to vent their own anger and to get revenge on their children; to enhance their own self-image by pushing their children down and labeling them as blameworthy (the parents can then uphold themselves as better than and above their children); to teach the children proper behavior.

Punishments are not the cure-alls many parents think them to be. They are more effective the less often they are used. Infrequent, occasional punishment does not significantly harm the parent-child relationship. The most important danger of punishment is not its occasional use but its overuse.

Excessive reliance on punishment has several undesirable effects.

The child fails to develop self-control, because punishment is a form of external control. His psychological brake pedal is provided by an outside source; thus he does not strengthen his ability to develop his own brake pedal. In fact, self-control is weakened by the overuse of punishment, and children who are punished often usually continue to misbehave.

The development of a sense of conscience is retarded when parents use too much punishment; instead self-centeredness and what's-in-it-for-me attitudes motivate the child, so that he becomes more concerned about being caught than about the wrongfulness of his actions.

Excessive punishment creates an automatic desire for revenge in the child, a wish to regain his sense of equality with his parents. He desires to get even with them, to hurt them in return for the hurt that he has experienced in being punished.

The child learns to lie in order to escape punishment. Some children develop a great talent for deception, and the more their parents punish them, the more skilled they become at lying and not being caught. Parents who use excessive punishment train their children to be skilled liars while failing to stop or reverse their patterns of misbehavior.

The child's self-esteem is severely harmed when parents use punishment excessively. He learns to think of himself as unworthy and deserving of the punishment and suffering. He may develop a sense of defeatism, of always doing things incorrectly and conclude that he is constantly in trouble. Because he feels that way, he may decide there is no point in improving his behavior. Gradually he may come to feel less loved, less appreciated, and less wanted within the family and, ironically, will often deliberately misbehave in order to obtain status, a place in the family, and a sense of identity. Excessive punishment, therefore, tends to create the very problems that parents wish it to destroy.

When punishment is used most effectively, it is used sparingly as a last-resort demonstration of the firm limit the parents have set on the child's misbehavior.

Punishment as a disciplinary technique should not be confused with logical consequences, which are more powerful and more effective; they are discussed in Chapter 13.

Help Your Child Find Legitimate Expression

Once ineffective methods are abandoned, you are free to use new, more powerful techniques. An important early step is to help your child find avenues of self-expression that will help him articulate his wants in an acceptable, socially useful manner. Your child will then no longer need to indulge in misbehavior to get his message across. Help your child transform his misbehavior into actions that will achieve his purpose without negative effects on others.

If your child throws things at his brother or sister when angry, teach him to ask them to stop doing or saying the things that he is angry about. Your intervention helps your child transform his physical misbehavior into a socially effective verbal outlet expressing his feelings and wants. A similar improvement would occur by teaching your child to say "I would like you to pay attention to me now," rather than misbehaving in order to convey the same message. Of course, your child must receive an honest and responsive answer to his requests if he is to learn to express his wants verbally rather than by his usual misbehavior.

Provide physical outlets to substitute for misbehavior. A mattress for bouncing and a pillow or punching bag for hitting can be effective. Toys for active play are discussed in Chapter 14. Recognize the importance of your child's needs by creating socially acceptable channels for their expression.

Surrender Your Need to Control

Making behavior choices within the limits you set gives him a sense of personal influence in the situation and helps to develop his initiative and self-control. If crayons need to be put away, for example, allow your child to choose when to do it within the hour.

Your child should be allowed to develop his own style and unique way of doing things. There is danger in pressuring him not only to do it, but to do it now, your way, perfectly, better than others, and so forth.

As long as your child is not jeopardizing his own welfare, violating the rights of others, or ignoring a principle that is necessary for maintaining order in the situation, there is little need for imposing disciplinary techniques. At these times strengthen the love bond between you in ways that do not involve discipline by talking and playing with him, giving instruction and guidance, and being a companion to him.

Negative feelings, expressed appropriately through legitimate channels, improve the relationship. Do not be afraid of your child's occasional desire to express negative feelings about your actions. In turn, be willing to disclose your own negative feelings to him. Such an exchange of potentially hurtful information must be done carefully and in a loving spirit. It is unfair and harmful for your child to learn to suppress his negative feelings out of fear that he will be rejected or punished if he expresses them.

Take Time for Training

Be willing to take advantage of every opportunity to teach important lessons to your child. Be willing to put yourself through temporary inconvenience for the greater purpose of teaching an important principle. Take actions that will help prevent future misbehavior. Turn around and come home from that trip; cancel that scheduled treat; stop the car until your child stops misbehaving in the back seat.

Don't wait until the stress situation occurs to start training your child. A visit with friends is not the time to start teaching your child how to behave when company is present. Dining at a restaurant is not the moment to start teaching table manners. Teach appropriate skills when you have enough time and energy to do it right. Don't rely solely on instant disciplinary techniques to teach your child while he is misbehaving in a provocative situation.

Maintain Firmness

Firmness means not permitting a violation of your own rights and is an excellent method for teaching your child to respect others' rights. Concern for others is the basis for the development of conscience.

Your child's natural tendency is to try to find out what works for him in life. He wants to explore the boundary of his power, and will push others as far as possible to make them be the way he wants them to be. Do not blame him for this natural desire.

Guide your child in how to be assertive in constructive ways, such as by defending himself against unfairness from others, stating his wants politely at family meetings, and making his requests to others clear and simple. Urge him to share his talents and skills with others, so that he can display his skills in positive, happy situations based on mutual enjoyment and cooperation.

Assert your own rights in a nondomineering, nonaggressive way, setting an example that permits your child to find out how he can legitimately find and exercise personal power. If you are weak, he will be terror-stricken as his natural quest for a sense of personal power forces him to trample you under a barrage of misbehavior. If this point is reached, your child will desperately want you to set limits to his actions. He will continue to push you in an attempt to force you finally to stand up and say "No more." Until you do this, he will pose the question: "How long are you going to let me do this to you?" By setting that firm limit, you will have reestablished your leadership of your child.

Use Misbehavior As a Clue to Unmet Needs

Misbehavior is a symptom of unmet needs. Thus it is a blessing as well as a curse, because it can steer you toward needed improvements and modifications in family life. Constantly keep in mind the goal of helping your child feel loved and helping him learn how to return that love.

His purposes for misbehaving can be understood in terms of his relations with other family members as well as their immediate social usefulness for him.

The Family Constellation—Birth Order and Sibling Rivalry

Your child's conception of himself comes from his awareness of others' traits and from comparing himself with others. How your child perceives his place within the family is a key to his self-esteem, and his interpretation of his place within the family is based in part on his reaction to the sequence in which children have come into your family.

His reaction to this birth order helps mold his awareness of methods for finding personal power and acceptance within the family. Sibling rivalry and birth order vary in their impact on family members, combining with other factors to contribute to your child's choice of actions at any specific moment.

Learn how your child perceives his position within the family in terms of birth order and you will be better able to recognize the purposes of his misbehavior. Until you know the purposes, you will not know how to suggest a substitute action that will achieve as much for him as his misbehavior will.

If the hyperactive child is your eldest, he may feel a need to maintain superiority over the second child. He may want to be first in everything. Perfectionism and excessive ambition may make him a prime candidate for eventual discouragement and frustration which can lead him to give up trying.

The process of seeing himself as dethroned by the second child may be painful for a hyperactive oldest child. He may try to regain what he considers his rightful place as the center of the family's interest. If the second child shows signs of achieving successes, the hyperactive oldest child may misbehave in order to keep the attention of the parents on himself. If the second child is quite successful in many areas, the hyperactive oldest child may surrender his oldest child status to his competitor and become irresponsible so that the burdens of being the oldest, such as being expected to be successful at school, fall upon his sibling's shoulders rather than his own.

If the hyperactive child is the second child, he may sense his failure at never quite measuring up to the first child, concluding that he always receives diluted love and attention from his parents because the oldest child receives the limelight. He may feel unworthy to have new clothes because he has always had to wear hand-me-downs from the oldest child. He may seem to be in a continuous race with the oldest child but may act uncertain of his abilities. He may try to become very different from the first child, to the point of being a polar opposite. If the older sibling is successful, the hyperactive second child may assume the role of being a failure. If the oldest child is well-mannered, the hyperactive second child may become the family brat.

If the hyperactive child is the youngest, he may feel as if he is in a foot race in which he must overtake the pack. You may notice that he seems to be climbing over people and manipulating them for his own gain. He may learn how to get family members to pamper him, wait on him, and rescue him from difficulties. Particularly if he has problems with coordination, he may develop the ability to get others to do things for him and to make decisions and accept responsibilities that should belong only to him.

Whatever the birth order sequence of your family and your child's place within it, how he perceives his relationship to siblings and parents determines to some extent his choice of behavior patterns. Misbehavior reflects his perception of and his response to his most desperate needs: attention because he fears being overlooked, power because he fears being overpowered.

The Four Goals of Interpersonal Misbehavior

Misbehavior achieves certain social gains for your child. It is not simply the result of accident or chance. It has purpose. Dr. Rudolph Dreikurs* was the first to formulate the four mistaken goals or hidden purposes of children's interpersonal misbehavior. The explanation of the four goals given here is an adaptation of his original concept.

The four mistaken goals of interpersonal misbehavior among children are: to obtain attention; to display power; to obtain revenge; to claim exemption from responsibility by assuming disability and inadequacy.

● GOAL I. SEEKING UNDUE ATTENTION. The most common purpose of children's misbehavior is to seek unwarranted and excessive attention and service from others. There are four types of attention-getting misbehavior:

1. *See what I can do!* This type involves a show-off egotistical style in which the child parades his accomplishments and fishes for praise. Parents usually become disgusted with the child's selfish attitude and scold the child for his egotism.
2. *Consider me special:* The child may come to expect special treat-

---

* Rudolph Dreikurs, M.D., was a child psychiatrist who trained under Alfred Adler and who later popularized many modern principles of parent-child relationships such as the family council, consequences rather than punishment in response to children's misbehavior, the importance of encouragement to children's self-esteem, and related notions. Some of his books are listed under Suggestions for Further Reading in the Appendices.

ment and exemptions, especially if he has been overprotected or is receiving medication or special foods. He may learn to manipulate others with smiles and charm, and conclude that he has a right to extraordinary treatment because he is different in a superior way from other children. He may appear angelic to his parents, who might simply be manipulated by his charm, but if sibling rivalry is involved, he usually claims an exalted status by being more angelic than his brother(s) or sister(s).

3. *Be occupied with me:* This pattern involves being a nuisance, whining, having tantrums, and being a brat. His parents usually react by feeling annoyed, bothered, and harassed. They want to shoo him away, and repeatedly tell him to stop misbehaving. Usually they feel like punishing, scolding, or criticizing him. He manipulates his parents into giving him lots of attention, but of a negative kind.

4. *Do it for me:* This type of attention-getting pattern is more common among young hyperactive children than among older ones, because the muscle control and coordination skills of young hyperactive children are usually not as developed as those of their playmates and classmates. The child is sloppy and appears lazy, negligent, or ignorant. He may procrastinate, ask to be reminded, expect to be cleaned up after. He manipulates others into doing things for him that he could do for himself. He manages to be waited on by parents and siblings because he appears helpless and asks others to serve him. Parents usually dislike being treated like slaves and resent being tricked into having to nag and remind so often. They become disgusted with the child's apparent helplessness.

When parents set limits on Goal I misbehavior by using stop-gap methods such as too early ignoring, punishment, piggyback messages, witchhunts, or parent tantrums, the child will usually stop the misbehavior for a brief period of time. A short while later, however, the misbehavior will very likely reoccur.

What to Do: Try to guide your child toward having a constructive impact on others. Help him learn to cooperate, to contribute unselfishly to others, and to be concerned with others' needs rather than just his own interests. Help your child be kind to others by making him aware of how good others feel as a result of his benevolent actions.

There can be a gradual change from forcing attention from others to affecting others in a positive and helpful way.

Support all benevolent, cooperative, and unselfish acts with encouragement. These acts are *not* to be used by the child to become better than others in the form of excessive goodness, but are to be used as experiences in learning how to live harmoniously with everyone who is part of his world.

Avoid giving piggyback messages. Substitute actions for words in responding in misbehavior of this type. The disciplinary methods discussed in Chapter 13 work well for transforming Goal 1 misbehavior into socially acceptable actions.

- GOAL II. DISPLAYING POWER. Another common goal of misbehavior is to invite power struggles and to attempt to dominate others. Because of their strong-willed nature, most hyperactive children display Goal II misbehavior on occasion. There are two patterns of power-displaying misbehavior, the active type and the passive type.

  1. *I'm the boss:* The active type involves out-and-out domination of others. The child is overwhelming and demanding. He must win and force others to submit to his will. Parents feel bullied, harassed, and defeated by the child's relentless pushiness.
  2. *Power struggle with me:* The passive type involves defiance and a contrary nature. The child is stubborn, rebellious, and sneaky. He wants to compete, oppose, and argue with others. There is a you-can't-make-me attitude, a chip-on-the-shoulder tendency to resist whatever others are trying to do or say. He experiences his power by opposing, and he does not have to win the contest in order to succeed in displaying his power. All he wants to accomplish is to put up a good fight.

In its early stages, Goal II misbehavior may be a testing process in which a simple, calm firmness from parents is quite adequate to stop the pattern. In a full-blown power display pattern, parents usually feel provoked, attacked, and challenged by the child. Often they conclude that their ability to influence him is being threatened and that their status and prestige are being attacked. A common first impulse is to force the child to change his actions and not to allow him to get away with such a challenge. By responding in this way, parents duplicate what the child is doing and make the situation worse. Whenever their power is challenged, they must overwhelm him with a greater display of power. When this happens, a terrible power struggle between parents and child begins. When parents respond with a stop-gap discipline technique, the child's misbehavior is immediately intensified. He digs in his heels, argues more energetically, and does almost exactly the opposite of what his parents want him to do.

What to Do: The right approach to the child who is trying to display power is to guide him toward cooperatively influencing others. Rebelliousness can become leadership and stubbornness can become determination to do what is socially useful and constructive. Self-discipline and self-sufficiency can replace the you-can't-control-me attitude. Once he has the self-confidence to experience personal power without needing to defend it excessively, he can allow others to influence him and can become more flexible and cooperative.

Because your child does not experience sufficient personal power, he makes a major effort to prevent anyone else from influencing him. You must withdraw from potential power struggles. At the same time, give your child opportunity to experience his own power by making legitimate small choices. His desire for power and influence over himself and others needs to be channeled into acceptable, legitimate avenues.

Stay calm, and encourage negotiation between the two of you. Recognize his potential power and skills. Avoid any invitation to continue the power struggle. Take the child aside and talk openly about the fact that you don't want to get into a needless power struggle with him. State plainly what you wish him to do, and state the ways in which you are willing to meet him halfway on the issue. Power struggles are prevented with kindness, never with force.

* GOAL III. GETTING REVENGE. The child who has this goal commits antisocial and destructive acts, appears bitter and negative about life, openly criticizes and rejects others, and tries to make his parents feel hurt and guilty by pointing out their errors and faults. He is trying to get even with the world by harming and punishing others. He may claim that he hates certain people and he may believe that the world owes him a favor in return for each difficulty that he experiences.

Parents usually feel rejected and confused about the child's bitterness. Their first impulse is often to get revenge on the child, to punish him, or to scold and criticize him. This first impulse is a mirror-image of what the child is doing to them. When they act on it, the way is open for a revenge struggle that can develop into a small-scale war. The child's response to stop-gap discipline techniques is simply to increase the misbehavior and attempt to get greater revenge on his parents.

What to Do: The child who tries to get revenge feels deeply hurt by others. Find and eliminate the underlying sources of your child's hostility. Talk with him at quiet moments, such as at bedtime. Make a special appointment to be alone with him if necessary. Explain that you realize how hurt and angry he must feel, and express a desire to improve the situation. As with power struggles, kindness rather than force is the only way to break the revenge cycle.

Your child needs to learn to respond to unkind deeds of others in a benevolent rather than in a revengeful way. Teach him the art of forgiveness and the value of kindness as responses to the unkind acts of others. Teach him to leave the situation if others are starting to act unkind, rather than staying and participating in further misdeeds or violence. Help your child learn that he can afford to be kind to others and that being kind is an act of strength, not weakness. Demonstrate this principle in your own dealings with others. Withdraw from others' unkindness; forgive and seek to repair the situation later.

• GOAL IV. ASSUMING DISABILITY AND DISPLAYING INADEQUACY. This type of misbehavior represents the greatest amount of personal discouragement in the child. In the other three types, the child is still fighting for what he needs and wants. In this type, he has given up.

The child's purpose is to be considered exempt from responsibility and participation. He has lost the desire to try any more. He concludes that he is unable to meet the expectations and demands of the situation. Like an opposum, he becomes absent or plays dead. He maintains a role of complete helplessness as a way of saying: "I can't do it; leave me alone." He is afraid to try new things and gives up on current projects, no longer contributing to the group or the activity. He claims special exemption because of his assumed incompetence, assumed personal inadequacy, or dislike for the activity or task, displaying an I-don't-care attitude about almost everything.

The child who is showing Goal IV misbehavior is afraid to risk the chance of making mistakes. He is usually terrified at the possibility of being recognized as imperfect. Rather than risking imperfection by giving an earnest try at a challenging task, the child excuses himself from the obligation to participate. The Goal IV child is a perfectionist, and like all perfectionists is unable to meet his own standards.

Parents usually feel baffled, frustrated, and desperate because the child rejects assistance and urgings. The first impulse is to coax, reassure, and persuade the child to participate. As the child continues to be passive and to expect exemption, they may become angry and critical toward him. As the process continues, they may throw their hands up in despair, finally giving up trying to get the child to participate. When this happens, he will have achieved his goal of truly being declared exempt. The parents will have illustrated the very pattern that they had been trying to uproot: they, too, will have given up and avoided the responsibility of dealing with the child's underlying personal discouragement.

When stop-gap discipline methods are used in response to Goal IV misbehavior, the child may become more firm in his determination to be declared exempt. He becomes even less willing to listen to his parents, less responsive to urgings, and less interested in taking initiative. This pattern often continues even though he may know that it is self-destructive. A typical example is failing to do school work even though he is aware of the value of getting an education.

What to Do: Building self-esteem is the most important part of overcoming a Goal IV pattern of misbehavior. The child who has given up needs a great deal of encouragement. The methods for displaying an encouraging attitude discussed in Chapter 5 are especially helpful. Uproot your child's fear of making mistakes. Display a constructive attitude toward your own mistakes, so that you illustrate an acceptance of being imperfect. Openly acknowledge your child's contributions and strengths.

Help him find constructive means of withdrawal. Teach him that withdrawal is for the purpose of renewal and preparation for further tackling of stressful situations. Help him recognize the value of temporary time-outs from stress in the form of breaks, vacations, holidays, and rest periods. Your child must learn how to slow down without actually stopping or giving up.

Promise yourself that you will not adopt Goal IV: do not give up your project of helping to lift your child out of the mire of complete discouragement. Don't let him continue to assume that he is completely incompetent, and be unimpressed by his attempt to display his inadequacy.

Chapter 13

Using More Effective Disciplinary Approaches

Taking preventive measures will help to reduce the instances of your child's misbehavior but there will still be times of conflict. Having discarded the five common inefficient disciplinary methods, you are now ready to use more effective techniques.

Natural Consequences

Natural consequences do not involve intervention by other people. They are the natural sequence of events after the child misbehaves. They are not manufactured by parents; instead they are simply allowed to occur. The natural consequence of your child's grabbing a small dog's fur is being nipped by the dog; of running on an icy sidewalk, a skinned knee; of experimental puffing on a cigar, coughing and choking; of grabbing playmates' toys, being rejected by playmates. Natural consequences are spontaneous ways of learning about life and can be powerful teachers.

When you want a natural consequence to become a corrective influence on your child, do not intervene. Temporarily divorce yourself from the situation as much as possible and be patient and quiet. Be your child's ally and avoid giving I-told-you-so speeches afterward. If he brings the event up for discussion, express hope that he will change his actions in some way next time so that things work out more pleasantly for all concerned. Treat the experience as you would any mistake—an opportunity to learn and improve.

In many instances, however, a natural consequence would not be the most efficient learning method. It might take too long to materialize, or it might jeopardize the child's health or safety. Sometimes an overriding concern, such as financial cost, must be given consideration. For example, the natural consequence of allowing a bicycle to stay out in the rain, is that it will rust; however, losing the use of his bicycle in that way may cause too much disruption to your child and to the family. The natural consequence of his coming to the table with dirty hands is that he may become ill, and the natural consequence of his playing carelessly in the street is that he may be hit by a car. Obviously adult intervention is needed in these instances.

Logical Consequences*

When it seems inappropriate to permit a natural consequence, you can intervene in a humane, sensitive, and loving way. The consequence of the misbehavior can be logically related to it.

Explain to your child the new actions you will take in response to his misbehavior. Communicate what you will do, and let your child decide what he will do. After your initial explanation, there is no need for piggyback messages about your new policies. Use logical consequences without continuing to explain or justify them to him.

When your child starts to misbehave, put the emphasis on controlling yourself rather than on controlling him. Stop cooperating with him. Don't do him any favors relevant to the misbehavior. In this way you can let him know that you do not endorse his misbehavior. Control what you will give to, do for, or permit for your child. Wash only those items of his clothing which he has placed in the correct laundry containers. Do not allow a plate for the child who comes to the table with dirty hands until they are washed.

Logical consequences are known ahead of time by all concerned. You guide them and he experiences them as logical in nature. If the conflict involves your child's tracking in mud, you can inform him ahead of time that he is to leave his muddy shoes on the porch from now on or he will have to mop up the kitchen if mud is tracked in.

Set a time limit for your child's combined work and play. Let him determine how much time he will have left to spend at play by the amount of time he takes to do his work. The longer he takes to do the dishes, for example, the less time there will be for you to be available for reading a story, because both activities must be accomplished by bedtime. The more your child delays you by badgering you about

---

* The first clear differentiation between natural and logical consequences was made by Maurice Bullard in 1963, in collaboration with Dr. Rudolph Dreikurs, who popularized both concepts.

something, the less time you will spend playing with him afterward. The longer he delays his bedtime preparations, the less time you will spend tucking him in.

A guideline should be: work must come before play. Prohibit play until his chores are done. If work is done before play, he will enjoy both activities more than if he had reversed the sequence. Work will be done quickly because he will be eager to begin his play, which he will enjoy more because he will have earned it. "You may go out to play after you have done the dishes and I have looked at them" and "As soon as you show me that your homework is done, you may watch television" are typical rules you set down.

Withdraw a privilege he abuses and give him a chance to regain it later when he shows that he can handle it responsibly. For example, temporarily deny him the use of his bicycle if he rides it carelessly, or forbid his use of the telephone temporarily if he has not used it properly.

Let the consequence do the teaching. Do not insist or even expect that he accept the consequences in any specific attitude or any special style. He might react to the consequence in any of a variety of ways: he might be angry, he might be quiet, he might pout, or he might show an attitude of resignation to it. The benefits can be lost if you become emotionally involved with his style of accepting the consequence.

It is important that logical consequences be used firmly, dramatically, quickly, and calmly. Your child should not be given a second chance or an opportunity to manipulate his way out of facing the consequence at the time of his misbehavior. You should remain firm and consistent without feeling guilty or sorry for him. The consequence should be fair, humane, justified and not delivered with vengeance. When a similar situation occurs in the future, your child will have another opportunity to choose a better course of action. "Next time you'll have another chance" is sufficient in response to any plea your child may make for a second chance.

Although logical consequences will not make you the helpful ally that you could be when you allow natural consequences, you will at least not be the adversary that you become when authoritarian punishments are used. Remain calm and exercise your parental responsibility of putting your child in touch with his strength and decision-making ability. Do not take actions that would make your child feel worthless, incapable, or unacceptable. You should never label him as bad or react to him with impatience or an urge for revenge or retaliation. Never rub things in with I-told-you-this-would-happen speeches. Make him aware that you do not enjoy his discomfort, and show empathy with his feelings of dismay. Your proper attitude should be one of mild regret that he has chosen to act in a way that has led to these consequences.

Even the most effective logical consequences can deteriorate into authoritarian punishments through misapplication. Coaxing, threatening, giving piggyback reminders, trying to force the situation, or failing to have a prior discussion about the consequences can destroy their effectiveness.

Table 4 lists some key points of contrast between logical consequences and authoritarian punishments.*

Logical consequences are generally more effective in response to Goal I misbehavior (seeking undue attention and service) than in response to the other misbehavior goals. Particular care must be taken with Goal II misbehavior (displaying power) because sometimes logical consequences can fuel a power struggle.

Therapeutic Affection

Many parents of hyperactive children report outstanding success from giving a large dose of pure affection at the start of misbehavior, before the situation gets out of control. The affection can be offered where and when the misbehavior occurs or during a time-out period in your child's room. An attempt at therapeutic affection should not be made when you are angry; it should be given early in the event, before you have built up negative feelings.

Often it can be given by holding your child on your lap or by sitting beside him. Gentle rocking or caressing the child also helps. Whisper a soothing comment such as: "I know that this is a rough time for you, and I don't want you to feel so upset." Let the conversation wander as you hold or affectionately touch him.

Sometimes a child will not like to be touched or held. In that case,

* Based in part on Dreikurs and Grey, 1968

TABLE 4   Logical Consequences vs. Authoritarian Punishments

Logical Consequences	Authoritarian Punishments
Express needs of the entire social situation	Express the power of the punisher
Logically related to the misbehavior	Arbitrary connection between misbehavior and punishments
Focus on present choices	Focus on the past
Involve encouragement of the child's self-esteem	Involve discouragement of the child's self-esteem
Resentment by the child is minimal, aimed at his own poor choices	Resentment by the child is great, aimed at the parent
Develop self-discipline	Depend on external authority for control of child's actions
Develop conscience, awareness of others' needs and rights	Do not develop conscience; child is concerned with his own pleasure and not getting caught
Do not humiliate the child	Often humiliate the child
Freedom of choice within limits	No choice is available to the child
Thoughtful and deliberate	Often given impulsively
Choice given only once	Often involve piggyback messages
Parent does not have a tantrum	Parent often has a tantrum
Parent controls his or her own actions	Parent tries to control all of the child's actions
Parent is not negatively involved with the child	Parent usually is negatively involved with the child
Imply that the child can make wise decisions	Imply that the parent must make decisions for the child

find a soothing activity that your child can enjoy, such as sitting near you or going for a walk together.

At one level or another, a child's misbehavior can be regarded as an appeal for love. Providing affection in a direct and generous way at the beginning of his misbehavior leaves him with no further purpose or interest in misbehaving. Therapeutic affection given in the manner outlined here will not reward the child for misbehaving and will not train him to misbehave every time he wants more love from parents. It will have the opposite effect. Your child will learn to ask you directly and openly for your affection and attention when he is needy, rather than misbehaving in order to force you to give him your love and attention.

Restructuring the Situation

Sometimes rearranging the location of people and objects will stop misbehavior. Other methods, such as therapeutic affection, can then be used to prevent future misbehavior.

Sometimes you may have to move your child into a new location to give him a chance to adjust his approach to a conflict situation. Introduce this restructuring arrangement with a statement such as: "It looks as if you are not ready to enjoy being here now." Physically escort your child to a temporary new location, such as his bedroom, and stay with him during this time-out period if necessary. He should need only a few minutes to regain his composure and get ready to try it again with a minor adjustment in his behavior.

Removing the audience for his misbehavior can sometimes eliminate the problem. If you are the entire audience, leaving the scene when your child displays Goal I misbehavior will drain it of its attention-getting power. Your withdrawal is not weakness; it is a strong statement of your firmness in not honoring the misbehavior by providing an audience for it.

Sometimes it may be necessary to remove objects that your child is playing with inappropriately. Remove a ball that he is throwing in the living room or any toy that he plays with in a dangerous or annoying manner. Use the event as a teaching opportunity, returning the object to your child after he has had a chance to reconsider how to use it.

If your child is completely out of control in a dangerous situation, you will have to restrain him physically. Approach him from behind, so that your stomach is pressing against his back. Stand behind him, cross his arms across his chest, and envelop him from behind with your arms. Maintain your grip until your child has calmed down and speak softly to him to lift him out of his frenzied state.

Just as a carpenter must have a variety of tools available in order to accomplish the goals of his trade, you must also have many tools and techniques available for your use in the most important job in the world—raising your children. No good carpenter would use a screwdriver in a situation that calls for a saw. In the same way, you must carefully select the disciplinary approach that best suits each situation. If you gradually decrease your use of the five inefficient methods of discipline mentioned in Chapter 12, you will notice that you will become calmer, more confident, and more effective as your child's leader. Good discipline is not harsh. By providing leadership without domination and influence without overcontrol, you can train your child in a positive way that maintains an atmosphere of mutual respect.

Chapter 14

Your Child at Play

A large part of your relationship with your child consists of the type of play experiences that you make available. Play, which occupies much of most children's days, teaches them a great deal about their social relationships, place within the family and peer groups, various academic skills, and numerous other talents that are useful throughout life. Play is, in some ways, children's work, providing opportunities for creativity and fantasy through pretending and for the discharge of large amounts of energy through movement and activity. The play activities of children have an important role in developing their innate capabilities into effective life skills.

Structuring Your Child's Play

Like any other aspect of your child's maturation, play activities require your intervention. Without becoming overinvolved, you can use play activities to help keep your child occupied and enrich his life. An important parental function is structuring, and sometimes supervising, your hyperactive child's play so that he has access to stimulating and wholesome means by which he can channel his energy and activity. It is unrealistic and nonproductive to put your child in the difficult position of having to use several consecutive hours of play time in random, haphazard actions merely to stave off boredom. He will benefit from play only if he is supervised to an appropriate degree.

Often the easiest way to help your child start a play activity is to arrange the setting ahead of time. Laying out the necessary materials and saying something like, "Here are some papers for you to cut out and put together," is better than asking him an open-ended question like, "What would you like to do now?" Give him an apron and some cleanup rags as part of the advance preparation if the activity involves the possibility of spilling things.

Group settings are generally more stimulating than solitary play for hyperactive children. Often a hyperactive child will do well for a limited period of time in group play but will gradually become overstimulated and bothersome to his playmates as the play time continues. Try to ease him into play groups for short periods of time at first. As his play becomes more cooperative, gradually increase the play time and the number of playmates. By careful observation you can determine how long your child can play with friends. End the play sessions before they deteriorate because of your child's increased excitability.

Integrating your child into group play activities is a rewarding but challenging task. Every so often observe the situation from a distance to achieve a balanced understanding of how he is getting along with other children. Listening only to your child's explanation of what went wrong with the play experience will give a one-sided picture. If he says, for example, "They won't let me play and they hit me and told me to get out," his statement may be true; however, he may not have reported what he was doing to aggravate his playmates in the first place. You can help your child best if you know exactly what aspect of his behavior the play group objects to.

Cooperative group play can work better if all of the children understand basic principles of courtesy. A few moments of supervision at the beginning of the play experience can provide the needed instruction. Teach your child, and the playmates if necessary, that possession of a piece of equipment is determined by its use—whoever is using it keeps it until finished with it. Throwing heavy or sharp-edged toys, taking toys apart, or any other act of destruction is not allowed. Pushing or hurting each other is forbidden. The children should be asked to take turns and to share.

Some of the principles of cooperative group play that your child must learn may seem several giant steps removed from his current form of play behavior. It is easy to become discouraged and frustrated at the hyperactive child's slow rate of improvement in learning to get along during play times. Unfortunately, parents usually show their disappointment more automatically and more vividly than they acknowledge their recognition of the hyperactive child's progress. Acknowledge his little gains and improvements, and be very specific in describing them to him. "It was very nice of you to let Billy take a turn right after you," emphasizes improvement while, "I see you still can't shoot baskets very well," stresses defeat. Many of the actions that can be lumped together as being a good sport are hard for a hyperactive child to understand. Such basic courtesies as waiting for his turn, sharing, talking politely, accepting without argument the fact that he is out for the moment, and appreciation of the skills of others may be difficult for your child at first. Under your specific instruction and supervision, however, your child can slowly develop good play habits which will serve him well throughout his life.

Your Child's Play Environment

Hyperactive children generally need a lot of space in which to move around, tumble, explore, run, and discharge their large amounts of energy. The hyperactive child who must live in an apartment without an adequate play area or who lives in a neighborhood without a large yard or nearby park or school playground may not be able to release enough energy. The result can sometimes be increased misbehavior and irritability, among other problems.

In addition to providing a large outdoor playing area, many parents of hyperactive children have found that a high fence or other protective partition helps assure them of the child's whereabouts and safety. The hyperactive child's unbridled curiosity and poorly developed sense of danger make some sort of physical barrier surrounding the play area even more necessary. Neighborhood improvements that increase the child's area for safe and free movement, such as sidewalks, are also desirable. In the country, hyperactive children usually enjoy roaming through large plots of land. Make sure that these open areas are safe to wander in.

Within the home, the hyperactive child needs a safe place for being very active. The best location would be a playroom in which the furniture is inexpensive and sturdy. It should contain various items for quiet as well as for active play. A corner can be set aside as a bouncing and tumbling place, created by placing one mattress on top of another on the floor. In a home without a playroom, a bouncing and tumbling place in a basement, attached garage, back porch, or other defined area will serve equally well.

Despite intentions to the contrary, most parents of hyperactive children find that the bedroom ends up being a playroom, too. Furnish the hyperactive child's bedroom with pieces that can stand heavy wear and tear and expect some physically rough treatment to the room and its contents through the years. The walls should be drab so that they do not overstimulate or frighten the child, especially at night; try to avoid loud and bright colors, stripes, and mirrors. The hyperactive child will probably need to have either the playroom or the bedroom as a time-out place for moments when he must be separated from others in order to reestablish cooperative behavior.

Your child should be encouraged to display his artistic creations. Arrange a place on a wall or shelf to show his work. Provide a set of shelves or drawers which are clearly labeled and easy to use, so that he can store his playthings without clutter.

The Importance of a Regular Family Play Time

In addition to the opportunity to play alone and the opportunity to play with other children, your hyperactive child needs to play with you. The importance of special parent-child play times cannot be overemphasized. It is crucial to increasing family harmony. At these times permit the child in you to respond to your child, so that a new and special bond can form, one that strengthens and expands the other types of loving and caring feelings that connect you with him. Parents who make a special place in their weekly schedule for a regular play time with their children usually find the experience surprisingly reassuring and fulfilling, even when other aspects of their relations with their children are not as positive or as pleasant.

Being able to have fun with your hyperactive child is essential to enjoying his company, regardless of any other feelings that you may have toward him. A regular play time has a number of other important rewards. It allows regularly available high-quality time for interacting with the child. It can be a pleasant change from conflict-laden types of interaction and can also counterbalance the less intense, watered-down experiences that occur when parents have busy schedules.

By allowing yourself to enter wholeheartedly into a play experience, you can temporarily abandon outside concerns and can focus on your home and family, using the opportunity to train your child in important skills.

Keeping a regular play time also permits you to give a fair share of yourself to your child. You can then do more things for yourself, your spouse, and the other children in the family without feeling apologetic or guilty. Regular play time also serves as a periodic reminder that fun is an important aspect of family life and of love for each other. Siblings will be far less jealous of the attention given to the hyperactive child if they know that they, too, have their own special place with you. Finally, regular play increases the loving feelings between you and your hyperactive child, strengthening the bonds of emotional caring, closeness, and mutual understanding.

Certain types of activities are much more beneficial than others at play time. In general, as discussed in detail in Chapter 9, games involving a winner against a loser in competition and rivalry are destructive and dangerous for the hyperactive child as well as the other children in the family. Cooperative games teach children the value of group effort and the importance of helping each other rather than trying to oppose and defeat each other.

One very helpful type of activity is playing together in situations that the child will face in the future. Giving a party, playing store, and similar experiences provide both rich learning opportunities and fulfilling forms of togetherness. Accompanying your child in active physical play such as climbing, digging, tussling, and organized sports can also be enjoyable. Just a casual walk with him through the neighborhood may provide an opportunity for genuine psychological intimacy.

Activities to Improve Your Child's Learning Skills*

In addition to providing entertainment, many activities can be instructional and can help build basic learning skills.

Auditory Skills

The abilities to hear well and to remember and organize what is heard can be strengthened by having your child close his eyes and try to identify the objects that you are holding by the sounds they make (toothbrush against cardboard, small electric motor, pencil on paper, etc.). Have your child try to find an object with his eyes closed, locat-

* Adapted from *Teaching Children with Special Learning Needs* by Milton Young (John Day, New York, 1967).

ing it by the sound that it makes (bell, whistle). Someone can wear a tinkling bell while your blindfolded child tries to catch him or her. A tape recorder, used under your supervision, can provide hours of entertainment and be an aid in self-expression.

Letter sounds can be used for many interesting activities. Riddle chaining is done by having your child make up a riddle whose answer starts with the last sound of the preceding answer. For example: "I say meow; what am I?" (ca*t*); "I am tall and have leaves; what am I?" (*t*ree); "I am a very thin fish; what am I?" (*ee*l).

Tell a story and leave out a word, pausing so that your child can fill in the correct and obvious word (" 'Twas the night before Christmas and all through the -----").

"Wouldn't it be funny if . . ." is a source of much amusement when the child takes turns with other family members in completing the statements with silly rhymes. ("Wouldn't it be funny if bees had fleas? . . . if sharks stayed in parks? . . . if flowers counted the hours?")

Say several words beginning with the same sound. Occasionally include a different beginning sound and have your child clap his hands when he hears the different sound.

Your child can tap out variations in rhythm and loudness that you first beat or tap out; handclaps are good to use for this entertaining exercise. While he has his eyes closed, have your child tell you how many times you have tapped with a pencil and on what object, or just have him identify sounds that he hears when sitting quietly.

Visual Skills

Have your child look carefully at a picture or drawing with a number of details in it; then have him draw it from memory, practicing until he can remember everything he sees in the picture.

Place several objects on a table; ask your child to turn away while you remove two of the objects; then have him try to guess what is missing.

Draw a picture but leave out one part; then let your child fill it in with crayon.

Using pictures of familiar objects, cut out one or two pieces from each and have your child identify what is missing and replace the missing parts.

Have your child join dots to form patterns of increasing difficulty;

[")}

then have him also draw letters, numbers, and objects that are outlined in dots.

Using two checkerboards, make a pattern with four checkers on your board and have your child duplicate it on his, gradually increasing the number of checkers. Eventually ask your child to try to duplicate the pattern from memory after he looks briefly at yours.

Have your child sort and arrange a collection of miscellaneous small objects by size, then by shape, color, and composition. Change the order in which pictures or objects are arranged, and have your child put them back in correct sequence.

Cover a word with a card; then slide the card slowly to the right so that the letters your child will read appear in proper sequence. Do the same for sentences, drawing the card so that words appear from left to right at a pace that is comfortable for your child. Make the sentences fun to read by including loving messages or humor in them.

Coordination

Construct a balance board by placing a board about two feet long on a horizontal cylinder, and have your child balance himself by placing his feet near each end of the board.

Play follow-the-leader as a family, and include lots of skipping, jumping, crawling, and use of right and left feet and hands.

Have your child walk while balancing a bean bag on his head or while pressing it between his knees; then have him hop, sit, lie down, or run with the bean bag in those positions.

Play charades as a family, acting out sentences, ideas or activities: going fishing, opening a jar.

Play "Simon Says" as a family, or play it with your child in front of a full-length mirror.

Do rhythms and dances as a family, such as stamping your feet, slapping your sides, Hokey Pokey, Farmer in the Dell, etc.

Have your child walk and skip backwards with you.

Have your child close his eyes and write in large letters on an extra-large sheet of paper or a small blackboard.

Cutting with scissors is an excellent activity. Start with large simple shapes and gradually have your child cut out more complicated and smaller shapes.

Ball and jacks is another good activity, as are large sewing cards.

Concept Formation

Start a scrapbook with your child. He can organize it into categories of his favorite things and collect pictures, news clippings, etc. about animals, sports, or other interests. At a simpler level, you can have your child categorize a collection of pictures of various objects (cut out of magazines) into appropriate subgroups, such as animals, plants, buildings, etc.

Memory games are also useful. "Going on a picnic or trip, I will take . . ." provides an entertaining activity for the entire family. Each person names all previously named items plus one more, so that the fifth person names the four previously mentioned objects in addition to adding a fifth object to the list.

Have your child memorize a short poem or nursery rhyme. Write it down and cut out the phrases; then scramble them and have your child replace them in order.

Guessing games also allow the development of concept formation ability. Have the child try to guess what object you are thinking of, providing only slight clues such as color or approximate size.

Having your child feel objects that are in a bag in order to guess what they are will also improve his ability at concept formation.

Guidelines for Selecting Toys

Your child's toys should require the involvement of as many senses as possible. He will enjoy toys that he can feel, move around, make sounds with, and which exercise his imagination. The complicated gadget that performs by itself while the child sits and looks at it is probably not a wise choice. He should be able to control the toy, rather than having the toy control him or operate without his participation.

Hyperactive children are usually attracted to items and activities involving self-expression rather than activities requiring focused or channeled concentration and restricted movement. Fingerpaints, modeling compound, guns that shoot small balls or darts, slimy semifluid, and confetti, for example, may be attractive to your child, while activities involving more restriction such as coloring books, small building pieces, table games, plastic target shooting machines, and plastic models may not seem attractive. However, the expressive items may be too limitless for your child and may serve to overstimulate him. Practice in focused attention is probably more beneficial in the long run because it is a skill that is useful at school and in adult life. You should strike a balance between toys that focus his attention and limit his responses and those that offer unlimited choices and great self-expression.

Toys for hyperactive children should be simple, durable, and safe. In many instances, it is better to provide a genuine item rather than a toy imitation. The added durability and realism of a genuine pocket radio, for example, make it preferable to a toy imitation radio. A small glider that really flies makes more sense than a heavy, out-of-proportion imitation of an airplane that can only roll on the floor.

Toys should not be fragile and should have little or no glass. There should be no pinching or cutting parts. Avoid electrical toys and those with lots of moving parts. Toys involving shooting or propelling hard or potentially dangerous objects should not be purchased.

These guidelines are very general, and allowance must be made for your child's own uniqueness and readiness for certain activities as well as for the play environment.

Some Toys for Quiet Play

Several types of useful toys for a hyperactive child's quiet play are artistic in nature. He will enjoy making art paper designs using blunt scissors, tape, or paste. In general, chalk and pencil are probably preferable to paint, ink, wax crayons, and felt markers. Although chalk creates dust, it is only a temporary nuisance and can easily be washed from clothes and walls. Paint-with-water books, in which the paint is already in the paper and just has to be brushed with water, avoid the hazards of using real paint while providing your child with the experience of painting.

Modeling clay and modeling dough can be meaningful forms of expressive play. (The artificial colors in these products, however, may create problems for hyperactive children who are sensitive to them.) You can use cookie cutters, rolling pins, and other utensils to help your child make things from these materials.

Art projects should allow for quick success and easy completion, for the hyperactive child is not a patient worker. For example, snap-together assembly will usually be a wiser choice than glue-together assembly of plastic models. After any art project is completed, your child may suddenly lose interest in it unless his work is displayed on a wall or shelf. As time goes on, you can encourage your child to use more care and have more patience with art projects.

Sets of tiny people are often useful. Puzzles that can be solved with a pencil can provide pleasant and educational entertainment. A sandbox can be a haven for writing, digging, and building. Small metal cars and trucks are good toys for sand and dirt play. For the young hyperactive child, the sturdy wood and plastic toys geared for preschoolers may be useful. Wind-up and self-propelled vehicles, such as small motorcycles and racing cars, can also be fun. Jigsaw puzzles should be matched to your child's abilities; the backs of the pieces can be color-coded to prevent any accidental mixing together of pieces from different puzzles.

Playing with some electrical toys may be enjoyable if supervision is provided. A record player, portable radio, walkie-talkie, or portable tape recorder might also be useful depending on your child's age.

Some Toys for Active Play

Many items can be stacked and used for building: cardboard or plastic blocks, cardboard boxes, plastic bowls with lids, margarine or food containers with lids, and oatmeal boxes. In general, commercially available wooden and plastic building toys have been found to be satisfactory for hyperactive children when matched to ability level and supervised.

Toys for punching and pounding that have been found to be appropriate for hyperactive children include sturdy punching bags, innertubes nailed to outdoor walls, and pillows. Some commercially available inflatable punching toys are not sufficiently sturdy to withstand the energetic and heavy use that a hyperactive child may give them.

Climbing, tunneling, and tumbling are important parts of your child's play needs, and such activities also tend to enhance his coordination. A large plastic trash can with holes cut in the sides can provide lots of fun. Supervise his play so that he doesn't get stuck. A simple tent made with bedspreads, sheets, or blankets draped over a card table or other piece of furniture can keep a hyperactive child happy. Large cardboard shipping cartons can become play caves but make sure there are air holes. Hopscotch markings chalked on cement and a basketball hoop placed low are aids in stimulating him toward play that will assist in the development of coordination.

Riding and moving toys may be useful. Plastic balls, plastic flying discs, and similar items can be used in safe and enjoyable lawn games.

With appropriate structure and supervision, water play can be an enjoyable experience for your child. Running through a sprinkler or playing with the hose on hot days can be fun. Squirt guns or unbreakable pitchers might also be allowed for water fights or similar games when supervision is available. Soap-bubble blowing can also be included as a pleasant indoor or outdoor activity.

Adolescent Recreation

The importance of your companionship increases after your hyperactive child reaches adolescence. Accompanying him to outdoor sporting activities or spectator games can be a mutually enjoyable experience, as can arts and crafts in which both of you participate.

Peer relationships are very important, and the hyperactive adolescent may want to participate in organized team sports. Often hyperactive children are not very successful at those sports, and sometimes have become so unpopular with their classmates and peers that they are not wanted on the teams. In such a situation, the adolescent needs help in regaining his popularity before he can enjoy this type of recreation.

Individual outdoor sports are generally preferred for the hyperactive adolescent over outdoor team sports. Activities such as running, swimming, biking, and skiing, for example, can develop his skills at a pace which is uniquely suited to his own readiness. There are no teammates to disappoint or seek approval from; there are no opponents to become angry at or feel inferior to. The adolescent competes against his own past record, striving for a faster or longer run, swim, etc. In this way, self-confidence can improve along with his level of skill.

Indoor recreation suitable for your child depends more on his personal preferences and habits than on the presence or absence of hyperactivity. Hyperactive adolescents enjoy table games if they are not too complicated and if there is not too much emphasis on competition. The mild activity offered by table tennis or billiards also seems to be attractive to hyperactive adolescents.

If this book emphasizes one theme, it is the necessity of nurturing and rebuilding the bonds of love in the family. Through play, regular meetings, companionship, guidance, observation of family members' actions, study of parent-child relationships, protection of the marital relationship, and a great deal of empathic understanding for the needs of each family member, love can be shown and experienced by the entire family. There can be no greater gift for the hyperactive child than to know he is loved, and none greater for his parents than to know that he has recognized their love for him.

APPENDICES

Appendix I

The Development of the Taylor Hyperactivity Screening Checklist

This checklist (see page 38) was developed from interviews with parents of hyperactive children. From these interviews, fifty-seven symptoms were gathered, and the list of these symptoms was given to parents of fifty-one hyperactive children. Each hyperactive child was from a different family, and their ages ranged from two to fifteen. All had been diagnosed as hyperactive by physicians and most were receiving medication treatment for hyperactivity. The parents rated their children on each of the fifty-seven traits and its matching opposite, using the same three-category system that appears on the checklist.

Twenty-one of the fifty-seven symptoms were selected for the final version of the checklist. These traits were those in which the children were rated in the hyperactive direction by at least 67 percent of the parents (thirty-nine out of fifty-one sets of parents), as well as those in which the children were rated in the nonhyperactive direction by less than 17 percent of the parents (three or fewer out of fifty-one sets of parents). In other words, those traits were very consistently rated in the hyperactive direction and were shown to be valid for screening hyperactivity.

The accuracy and validity of the checklist have been determined by administering it to various groups of children. A comparison of the results shows that it is highly accurate in screening out true hyperactivity from other conditions and from normal behavior. Table 5 shows the percentage of children rated showing each of the traits from the right side of the checklist, which are the hyperactive traits. The children are from four different groups. The first group contained fifty-one hyperactive children whose scores were used in developing the checklist. The second group contained sixty-six hyperactive children I saw in my professional practice in three years preceding the publication of this book. The third group consisted of twenty-two non-hyperactive siblings of the children from the first group. The fourth group consisted of nineteen children I saw in my professional practice who were not hyperactive but had other behavior difficulties.

Approximately four out of five hyperative children (81 percent and 82 percent for the two groups) were rated in the hyperactive direction on the checklist, while only one out of five nonhyperactive siblings without other

TABLE 5   Percentages of Children Rated in the Hyperactive Direction (Column C)

Item Number	Group 1 (51 hyperactive children)	Group 2 (66 hyperactive children)	Group 3 (22 nonhyperactive siblings)	Group 4 (19 nonhyperactive behavior-problem children)
1	82	79	23	26
2	82	71	14	32
3	78	79	18	37
4	82	77	9	32
5	92	91	32	47
6	76	82	14	21
7	82	89	32	53
8	92	91	23	53
9	94	92	41	58
10	71	70	32	32
11	88	91	16	42
12	82	82	36	42
13	78	70	23	11
14	86	91	36	47
15	76	70	14	37
16	80	68	9	42
17	84	79	23	47
18	90	86	32	68
19	88	86	14	58
20	76	70	9	21
21	67	82	18	42
Averages:	82	81	22	40

disorders (22 percent) were rated in the hyperactive direction. Of children with other behavior disorders only two out of five (40 percent) were rated in the hyperactive direction.

Another way to express these findings is to say that the checklist contains traits on the right side that occur in four out of five hyperactive children, but occur in only one of five siblings without disorders and two of five children with nonhyperactive behavior disorders.

Table 6 shows the percentage of children rated as showing each of the traits from the left side of the checklist, which are the normal opposites of the hyperactive traits.

Approximately three out of five nonhyperactive siblings without other disorders (61 percent) were rated in the nonhyperactive direction, while five out of ten (49 percent) of nonhyperactive children with behavior disorders were rated in the nonhyperactive direction. Fewer than one in eight hyperactive children (12 percent and 5 percent) were rated in the nonhyperactive direction. In other words, the traits on the left side of the checklist occur

TABLE 6   Percentages of Children Rated in the Non-hyperactive Direction (Column A)

Item Number	Group 1 (51 hyperactive children)	Group 2 (66 hyperactive children)	Group 3 (22 nonhyperactive siblings)	Group 4 (19 nonhyperactive behavior-problem children)
1	6	12	64	63
2	4	21	59	58
3	8	17	64	63
4	8	18	86	63
5	2	6	55	32
6	6	9	82	63
7	2	9	68	37
8	0	5	68	47
9	2	5	41	21
10	6	24	64	47
11	0	2	59	37
12	2	6	50	53
13	10	20	68	74
14	2	6	50	47
15	2	17	68	42
16	16	27	59	58
17	6	18	64	47
18	4	5	36	21
19	2	2	55	26
20	8	24	55	79
21	6	9	68	47
Averages:	5	12	61	49

in less than one in eight hyperactive children but occur in three of five non-hyperactive siblings without other disorders and in approximately one-half of nonhyperactive children with behavior disorders.

In summary, the hyperactive traits on the right side of the checklist appear to occur frequently in hyperactive children and rarely in nonhyperactive children. Their normal opposites on the left side appear to occur frequently in nonhyperactive children and rarely in hyperactive children.

Appendix II
Suggestions for Further Reading

Section One: The Trait of Hyperactivity
Wender, Paul: *The Hyperactive Child: A Handbook for Parents* (Crown, New York, 1973)

Section Two: Approaches to Treatment
Bosco, James and Stanley Robin: *The Hyperactive Child and Stimulant Drugs* (University of Chicago Press, Chicago, 1977)
Renshaw, Domeena: *The Hyperactive Child* (Little, Brown & Co., Boston, 1975)
Stewart, Mark and Sally Olds: *Raising a Hyperactive Child* (Harper & Row, New York, 1973)
Walker, Sydney III: *Help for the Hyperactive Child* (Houghton Mifflin, Boston, 1977)
Wender, Paul: *op cit.*

Readings on Additive-free Cooking and the
Feingold Nutritional Program
Crook, Dr. William G.: *Can Your Child Read? Is He Hyperactive?* (Pedicenter Press, Tennessee, 1975)
———— *Tracking Down Hidden Food Allergy* (Pedicenter Press, Tennessee, 1976)
Feingold, Dr. Ben: *Why Your Child Is Hyperactive* (Random House, New York, 1974)
Feingold, Dr. Ben and Helene: *The Feingold Cookbook for Hyperactive Children* (Random House, New York, 1979)
Goldbeck, Nikki and David: *The Supermarket Handbook: Access to Whole Foods* (Signet Books, New York, 1976)
Hunter, Beatrice Trimm: *Consumer Beware: Your Food and What's Been Done to It* (Bantam Books, New York, 1971)
Jacobson, Michael: *Eater's Digest: The Consumer Factbook of Additives* (Doubleday, New York, 1972)

Section Three: Feelings and Relationships in Your Family

Allred, G. Hugh: *How to Strengthen Your Marriage and Family* (Brigham Young University, Provo, Utah, 1976)

Briggs, Dorothy: *Your Child's Self-Esteem* (Doubleday, New York, 1975)

The Church of Jesus Christ of Latter-Day Saints: *Family Home Evening Manuals* (Salt Lake City, Utah, 1965 to present)

Corsini, Ray and Genevieve Painter: *Practical Parent: The ABC's of Child Discipline* (Harper & Row, New York, 1975)

Dinkmeyer, Don and Gary McKay: *Raising A Responsible Child* (Simon and Schuster, New York, 1973)

Dreikurs, Rudolph and Vicki Soltz: *Children: The Challenge* (Hawthorne, New York, 1964)

Dreikurs, Rudolph *et al: Family Council: The Dreikurs Technique* (Regnery, Chicago, 1974)

Fletcher, Judy: *Games: Activities for Your Christian Family* (Concordia, St. Louis, 1978)

Malterre, Martha: *Family Fun Time* (Awareness Education Seminars, 1978; available from Alfred Adler Institute, 159 N. Dearborn, Chicago, Illinois, 60601)

Nutt, Grady: *Family Time: A Revolutionary Old Idea* (Million Dollar Round Table, 2340 River Road, Des Plaines, Illinois, 60018, 1977)

Osman, Betty. *Learning Disabilities: A Family Affair* (Random House, New York, 1979)

Peairs, Lillian and Richard: *What Every Child Needs* (Harper & Row, New York, 1974)

Satir, Virginia: *Peoplemaking* (Science & Behavior Books, Palo Alto, California, 1975)

Stewart, Mark and Sally Olds: *op. cit.*

Section Four: Your Child At School

Baruth, Leroy and Daniel Echstein: *The ABC's of Classroom Discipline* (Kendall/Hunt, Dubuque, Iowa, 1978)

Canfield, Jack and Harold Wells: *One Hundred Ways to Enhance Self-concept in the Classroom* (Prentice-Hall, Englewood Cliffs, N.J., 1976)

Dinkmeyer, Don and Rudolph Dreikurs: *Encouraging Children to Learn: The Encouragement Process* (Prentice-Hall, Englewood Cliffs, N.J., 1963)

Dreikurs, Rudolph, Bronia Grunwald, and Floy Pepper: *Maintaining Sanity in the Classroom* (Harper & Row, New York, 1971)

Fairchild, Thomas: *Managing the Hyperactive Child in the Classroom* (Learning Concepts, 2501 N. Lamar, Austin, Texas 78705, 1975)

Gwinnett County Schools: *The Funtastic Book* (Lawrenceville, Georgia 30245, 1977)
Stewart, Mark and Sally Olds: *op cit.*

Section Five: Guiding Your Child
Corsini, Ray and Genevieve Painter: *op. cit.*
Dinkmeyer, Don and Gary McKay: *op. cit.*
Dreikurs, Rudolph and Loren Grey: *Logical Consequences: A New Approach to Discipline* (Hawthorn, New York, 1968)
Dreikurs, Rudolph and Vicki Soltz: *op. cit.*
Peairs, Lillian and Richard: *op. cit.*
Young, Milton, *Teaching Children with Special Learning Needs* (John Day, New York, 1967)

Appendix III

Questions and Projects for Group Discussion

Chapter 1: Is Your Child Hyperactive?
1. What are the three most meaningful sentences for you in this chapter?
2. What surprised you most in this chapter?
3. Which of the twenty symptoms occur most consistently in your child?
4. What might account for the apparently greater incidence of hyperactivity among boys than among girls?
5. What might account for the apparent decrease in hyperactivity during early adolescence in some hyperactive children?
6. What is your child's score and category on the Taylor Hyperactivity Screening Checklist?

Chapter 2: Counseling and Medical Treatment
1. What are the three most meaningful sentences for you in this chapter?
2. What surprised you most in this chapter?
3. Give examples from your experience of trying to be a facilitator of professional help for your child:
    a. when you were too insistent;
    b. when you were not insistent enough;
    c. when you were insistent without being pushy.
4. Why do I caution parents not to rush too quickly into medication treatment?

Chapter 3: Treatment by Nutrition Management
1. What are the three most meaningful sentences for you in this chapter?
2. What surprised you most in this chapter?
3. Give some indicators of the prevalence of food additives which are meaningful to you.
4. Select a typical daily menu for your child, and list all items which contain a potentially disturbing substance.
5. Of the advantages of this method of treatment, which are the most important for your situation?
6. Of the potential difficulties with this method of treatment, which are the most important for your situation?

Chapter 4: Treatment by Prescribed Medication
1. What are the three most meaningful sentences for you in this chapter?
2. What surprised you most in this chapter?
3. A common error is to discontinue medication when there appears to have been no change in the child's behavior after being given a low dosage of medication. What could be the reasons for the lack of improvement?
4. Of the advantages of this method of treatment, which are the most important for your situation?
5. Of the potential difficulties of this method of treatment, which are the most important for your situation?
6. Why do you suppose I have included nutrition management and counseling as well as medication as forms of treatment of hyperactivity?

Chapter 5: Your Child's Self-Esteem
1. What are the three most meaningful sentences for you in this chapter?
2. What surprised you most in this chapter?
3. Give examples of the presence of each of the seven major emotional stresses in your child.
4. Of the seven emotional stresses, which has been most severe for your child?
5. Contrast the approaches that you have seen other adults use with those given in this chapter for teaching your child to use mistakes wisely.
6. Apply at least three specific ideas from this chapter for one week and report results.

Chapter 6: Your Feelings About Your Child
1. What are the three most meaningful sentences for you in this chapter?
2. What surprised you most in this chapter?
3. Of the early physical stresses, which were most difficult in your situation?
4. Of the feelings of guilt and inadequacy, in which areas did you feel most responsible and/or inadequate?
5. Which of the five styles of overinvolvement exist the most in your relations with your child?
6. What have been some of your major fears and worries with regard to your family?
7. Pick out at least three specific recommendations from this chapter, apply them for one week, and report results.

Chapter 7: Your Child's Effect on Your Marriage
1. What are the three most meaningful sentences for you in this chapter?
2. What surprised you most in this chapter?

3. Pick out at least three of the methods listed for strengthening your marriage, apply them for one week, and report results.
4. Which of the twelve destructive marital patterns have occurred in your situation?
5. Cite an instance in which co-parenting would have prevented a difficult family experience.

Chapter 8: Your Child's Relations with Other Children
1. What are the three most meaningful sentences for you in this chapter?
2. What surprised you most in this chapter?
3. Which of the eight stress areas occur most consistently in your child's life?
4. Cite an instance in which other children may have had an interest in keeping your child upset and misbehaving.
5. How does a child's self-esteem affect his response to corrective messages from others?
6. Perform the wrist-slapping demonstration with an adult, and list the resulting teaching points about revenge.
7. Of the methods for decreasing sibling rivalry, which seem to be most potentially needed and useful in your situation?

Chapter 9: Rebuilding Family Harmony
1. What are the three most meaningful sentences for you in this chapter?
2. What surprised you most in this chapter?
3. Describe what can happen to a parent-child relationship when there is:
   a. too much love and not enough discipline;
   b. not enough love and not enough discipline;
   c. not enough love and too much discipline.
4. For each of the following, list at least three types of circumstances in which:
   a. you enjoy being with your child;
   b. your child enjoys being with you;
   c. your child enjoys doing something with your family;
   d. your family enjoys doing something including your child.
5. List at least three old habits that you must break in order to respond supportively to decreases in your child's hyperactivity.
6. Cite at least one instance from your family experience which illustrates that children misbehave in part because they fear there is not enough love to go around in the family.
7. Of the eight methods given for increasing the felt love in your family, which appear to be the most potentially useful for your family?

8. Apply one of the eight methods at least twice in one week, and report results.
9. Of the advantages listed for cooperative play, which seem to be the most important for helping your child?
10. Have at least four consecutive Family Council meetings according to the guidelines given in this chapter and report results.
11. Why do you suppose I emphasize the Family Council?

Chapter 10: Getting Help at School
1. What are the three most meaningful sentences for you in this chapter?
2. What surprised you most in this chapter?
3. Cite examples from your personal experience of truly helpful attitudes and approaches by a teacher.
4. Give examples from your personal experience of smooth cooperation among professional helpers in connection with your child's school adjustment.

Chapter 11: Effective Teaching Approaches
1. What are the three most meaningful sentences for you in this chapter?
2. What surprised you most in this chapter?
3. Of the suggested approaches for teachers to use, which ones seem most important for best assisting your child:
    a. in reading skill;
    b. in ability to focus attention and concentrate in class;
    c. in ability to get along with classmates.
4. Ask a cooperative teacher to read Chapters 10 and 11; then try to get an uncooperative teacher to do the same. Report results.

Chapter 12: Laying the Groundwork for Discipline
1. What are the three most meaningful sentences for you in this chapter?
2. What surprised you most in this chapter?
3. Write a statement to a hyperactive child explaining medication or nutrition management. Include the idea that such treatment may allow, but will not force, more appropriate behavior. Share it with the group.
4. Which of the preventive methods given in the first section of this chapter would be most helpful if vigorously applied in your situation?
5. Provide positive wordings as substitutes for these negatively worded directives:
    a. "Don't throw the ball in the living room!"
    b. "Don't eat so fast!"
    c. "Don't be selfish with your toys!"
    d. "Don't talk so loud!"

6. Although giving well-timed reminders may be helpful, what in general are pitfalls to be avoided in giving reminders?
7. Describe the process by which ignoring disrupts communication.
8. Describe examples of how you can personally tell when you are about to go on a witchhunt.
9. Describe the circumstances under which ignoring can most effectively be used as a discipline tool.
10. Cite at least three inefficient piggyback messages that you routinely give to your child.
11. Count the number of instances in which you give piggyback messages to your child on each of seven consecutive days, and report results.
12. Which of the five indicators of excessive piggyback messages occur in your family?
13. How does my statement about the primary function of discipline differ from other opinions that you have heard?
14. Of the family constellation stresses listed in this chapter, which seem to have occurred in your child?
15. Of the four mistaken goals of children's interpersonal misbehavior, which does your child appear to be seeking most often?
16. For each of the mistaken goals, I list several indicators. List the indicators that will help you discern whether your child is seeking Goal I (undue attention and service).

Chapter 13: Using More Effective Disciplinary Approaches
1. What are the three most meaningful sentences for you in this chapter?
2. What surprised you most in this chapter?
3. List at least five differences between:
    a. natural consequences and logical consequences;
    b. logical consequences and authoritarian punishments.
4. What are some potential drawbacks to relying on natural consequences as disciplinary measures?
5. Give therapeutic affection in an instance in which formerly you would have been tempted to become harsh toward your child, and report results.
6. Why does work before play serve as a better guideline than play before work?
7. List several ways in which a logical consequence can deteriorate into a less efficient method, if guidelines in this chapter are not followed.
8. Give several descriptive phrases that would portray the parent who applies the discipline strategy outlined in Chapters 12 and 13, e.g. quiet, firm, an ally to the child, etc.

Chapter 14: Your Child at Play

1. What are the three most meaningful sentences for you in this chapter?
2. What surprised you most in this chapter?
3. In what ways can play be considered an important activity for a child?
4. Of the methods of structuring and supervising your child's play, which seem to be most appropriate in your situation?
5. Of the recommendations given in this chapter, which appear to be the most fitting response on your part to your child's apparently slow progress?
6. Compare the structure and furnishings in your child's bedroom with those I describe as ideal.
7. Have a regular daily family play time for seven consecutive days, and report results.
8. List and share with other parents the types of toys that you have found to be appropriate for your hyperactive child:
   a. at quiet individual play;
   b. during active individual play;
   c. during active group play.

Appendix IV

Some Additive-Free Medicines

This list should not be regarded as inclusive of all available additive-free medicine. From time to time there are changes in composition of medicines, and new products become available which do not contain artificial ingredients. The counsel of the physician and pharmacist should be sought in order to arrive at the specific medicine best suited to the child.

In general, if a capsule is colored, only the white powder inside can be considered possibly additive-free. Some white medicines contain a small amount of dye, so the white color of the medicine is not a sure indicator of the absence of artificial ingredients.

NON-PRESCRIPTION MEDICINES

Antihistamines

Rhinosyn—antihistamine-decongestant, for 6 years and older

Rhinosyn DM—for runny nose with cough

Rhinosyn PD—antihistamine-decongestant for children with allergy symptoms

Rhinosyn X—for thick hacky cough with heavy mucus

For fever or pain

Acetominophen

Datril tabs

Oraphen liquid

Tylenol tabs

Valadol tabs

Other white tab forms of Acetominophen

For poison oak and poison ivy

Cortisone cream and lotion, ¼% and ½%

Sun screens

Pabafilm lotion

Pre-Sun lotion

PRESCRIPTION MEDICINES

For asthma

Alupent tabs

Brethine 2.5 mg. and 5 mg. tabs

Bricanyl tabs

Elixophyllin SR 125 mg. and 250 mg. caps (entire caps are o.k.) and 100 mg. caps (powder in caps)

Isuprel 10 mg. and 15 mg. tabs
Lixaminol syrup
Metaprel 20 mg. tabs
Quadrinal tabs
Slo-phyllin 100 mg. and 200 mg.
tabs and 60 mg. caps
Slo-phyllin GG caps
Slo-phyllin GG syrup (has lemon-
vanilla flavor)
Tedral and Tedral Expectorant
tabs, 25 mg. or SA tabs
Theo-dur tabs
Theophyll 225 mg. tabs
Theophylline generic (o.k. if white
pressed tabs)
Ventair tabs

For diarrhea and abdominal cramps
Donnatal tabs and powder in caps
Lomotil tabs (not for small chil-
dren)

For fever or pain
Acetominophen with Codeine
(white tabs)
Demerol tabs
Hycodan

For motion sickness
Marezine tabs

Antibiotics
Amoxicillin (powder in caps)
Ampicillin (powder in caps)
Cephalosporins (powder caps)
Anspor
Kefle)
Velosef

Clindamycin
Cleocin (powder in caps)
Erythromycin
Ilosone 125 mg. and 250 mg. caps
(powder in caps)
Lincomycin
Lincocin (powder in caps)
Penicillin G tabs
Penicillin G Potassium 400,000
unit tabs
Pentids 200,000 unit and
400,000 unit tabs
Pfizerpen G tabs
Penicillin V
Penapar VK 250 mg. and 500
mg. tabs
Penicillin VK tabs
Pen-Vee K 125 mg., 250 mg., and
500 mg. tabs
Pfizerpen VK 250 and 500 mg.
tabs
Robicillin VK 250 and 500 mg.
tabs
Uticillin VK 250 and 500 mg.
tabs
Veetids 500 mg. tabs
Penicillins, synthetic (powder in
caps)
Bactocil
Dynapen
Prostaphlin
Tegopen
Veracillin
Versapen
Sulfa
Bactrum DS tabs
Gantrisin tabs
Renoquid tabs (over age 14)
TAO caps
Tetracycline (over age 9) (powder
in caps)

Anticonvulsants
Celontin (powder in caps)
Clonopen 2 mg. tabs
Depakene (liquid in caps)
Dilantin Kapseals (powder in caps)
Mebral tabs
Mysoline 50 mg. and 250 mg. white
    tabs
Phenobarbital white tabs
Phenytoin caps
Tegretol 200 mg. tabs
Valium 2 mg. tabs
Zarontin (powder in caps)

Antifungal oral medicines
Griseofulvin
    Fulvicin tabs
    Grifulvin and Grifulvin V tabs
    Grisactin (powder in caps)
    Gris-Peg tabs

For poison oak and poison ivy
Cortisone creams, 1%

Antihistamines and deconges-
tants
Actidil 2.5 mg. tabs
Actifed tabs
Benadryl (powder in caps)
Brexin (powder in caps)
Co-Pyronil (powder in caps)
Fedahist white tabs
Isochlor time caps
Optimine tabs
Periactin 4 mg. tabs
Pyribenzamine with ephedrine tabs
Sudafed 60 mg. tabs
Vistaril (powder in caps)

Steroids, oral
Aristocort 4 mg. and 16 mg. tabs
Decadron 4 mg. tabs
Deltasone 5 mg., 10 mg., and 50
    mg. tabs
Dexone 4 mg. tabs
Gammacorten .75 mg. tabs
Hexadrol .75 mg. tabs
Hydrocortisone tabs (various
    brands)
Kenacort 1 mg., 2 mg., and 4 mg.
    tabs
Medrol, 4 mg., 16 mg.
Meticorten tabs
Prednisone tabs (various brands)
Sterane tabs

Miscellaneous medicines
Thyroid medicine:
    Letter .5 mg. tabs
    Armour Thyroid tabs
    Cytomel tabs
Diuretics:
    Diuril 250 mg. and 500 mg. tabs
    Lasix 20 mg. and 40 mg. tabs
For heart problems:
    Lanoxin .25 mg. tabs
For gout:
    Zyloprim 100 mg. tabs
For Parkinsonian condition:
    Artane 2 mg. and 5 mg. tabs
Tremin, 2 mg. and 5 mg. tabs
Fluoride:
    Fluoride drops (except with
        vitamins)
    Fluoride 2.21 mg. unflavored tabs

Appendix V

Feingold Associations

(as of March, 1980)

NATIONAL HEADQUARTERS

Feingold Association of the United
   States

Drawer A–G
Holtsville, NY 11742

REGIONAL HEADQUARTERS

Region 1:
Connecticut, Maine, Massachu-
setts, New Hampshire, Rhode
Island, Vermont
50 South Cogswell Street
Bradford, MA 01830

Region 2:
New Jersey, New York, Puerto
Rico, Virgin Islands
40 Buckbee Road
Troy, NY 12180

Region 3:
Delaware, District of Columbia,
Maryland, Pennsylvania, Vir-
ginia, West Virginia
13602 Crispin Way
Rockville, MD 20853

Region 4:
Alabama, Florida, Georgia, Kentucky, Mississippi, North Carolina, South Carolina, Tennessee
4652 Savage Creek Drive
Macon, GA 31210

Region 5:
Illinois, Indiana, Michigan, Minnesota, Ohio, Wisconsin
11221 West Lorry Lane
Minnetonka, MN 55343

Region 6:
Arkansas, Louisiana, New Mexico, Oklahoma, Texas
1308 Colony Road
Metairie, LA 70003

Region 7:
Iowa, Kansas, Missouri, Nebraska
812 North 17th Street
Blue Springs, MO 64015

Region 8:
Colorado, Montana, North Dakota, South Dakota, Utah, Wyoming
1988 South 700 West
Woods Cross, UT 84087

Region 9:
Arizona, California, Guam,
  Hawaii, Nevada
20310 Big Rock Drive
Malibu, CA 90265

Region 10:
Alaska, Idaho, Oregon, Washing-
  ton
P.O. Box 2031
Salem, OR 97308

OUTSIDE UNITED STATES

CANADA
Feingold Assn. of Durham
861 Finch Avenue
Pickering, ONT L1V 1J4

NORWAY
Feingold Assn. of Norway
Straumesvingen 40
N-5064, Norway

ALL OTHER COUNTRIES
International Liaison
Feingold Assn. of the United States
Drawer A–G
Holtsville, NY 11742

HEADQUARTERS WITHIN REGIONS

ALABAMA (Region 4)
FADA for Hyperactive Children
P.O. Box 1828
Dothan, AL 36303

Chattahoochee Valley Feingold
  Assn.
Route 5, Box 536
Phenix City, Al 36867

ALASKA (Region 10)
Regional Headquarters

ARIZONA (Region 9)
Feingold Assn. of Lake Havasu
  City
3411 Silver Saddle
Lake Havasu City, AZ 86403

Feingold Assn. of Phoenix Area
4727 S. Fairfield
Tempe, AZ 85282

Feingold Assn. of Yuma
Box 5812
Yuma, AZ 85364

ARKANSAS (Region 6)
Feingold Assn. of Jonesboro
3515 Viking, #B
Jonesboro, AR 72401

CALIFORNIA (Region 9)
Feingold Assn. of Monterey Area
P.O. Box 22884
Carmel, CA 93922

Feingold Assn. of Sacramento
4306 Glen Vista Street
Carmichael, CA 95608

Feingold Assn. of Southern Califor-
  nia
P.O. Box 1565
Fontana, CA 92335

Feingold Assn. of Fresno
P.O. Box 9861
Fresno, CA 93705

Glendora Chapter of Feingold
Assn. of Southern California
1125 E. Walnut Avenue
Glendora, CA 91740

Mid-Peninsula Chapter of Feingold
Assn. of the Bay Area
P.O. Box 1351
Los Altos, CA 94022

Malibu-Santa Monica Chapter of
Feingold Assn. of Southern California
20310 Big Rock Drive
Malibu, CA 90265

Feingold Assn. of Modesto
1445 Del Vale
Modesto, CA 95350

Feingold Assn. of Napa Valley
1211 Hagen Road
Napa, CA 94558

Alameda County Chapter of Fein-
gold Assn. of the East Bay
P.O. Box 787
Newark, CA 94560

Orange County Chapter of Feingold Assn. of the South Bay
2519 Dorothy Drive
Orange, CA 92669

Feingold Assn. of Northern California
6060 Gilbert Drive
Palo Cedro, CA 96073

Feingold Assn. of Redlands
P.O. Box 1183
Redlands, CA 92373

Feingold Assn. of the South Bay
P.O. Box 7000–136
Redondo Beach, CA 90277

Contra Costa Chapter of Feingold
Assn. of the East Bay
P.O. Box 55
Rheem Valley, CA 94570

Feingold Assn. of the Bay Area
P.O. Box 596
San Carlos, CA 94070

San Mateo Chapter of Feingold
Assn. of the Bay Area
P.O. Box 1212
San Carlos, CA 94070

Feingold Assn. of San Diego
1430 Morena Boulevard, Suite D
San Diego, CA 92110

San Francisco Chapter of Feingold
Assn. of the Bay Area
P.O. Box 16423
San Francisco, CA 94116

San Jose Chapter of Feingold Assn.
of the Bay Area
P.O. Box 8285
San Jose, CA 95155

Marin Chapter of Feingold Assn. of
the Bay Area
P.O. Box 944
San Rafael, CA 94902

Feingold Assn. of Sonoma County
5297 Gilchrist Road
Sebastopol, CA 95472

San Fernando Valley Chapter of
Feingold Assn. of Southern California
14134 Tyler Street
Sylmar, CA 91342

Feingold Assn. of the North Bay
71 "D" Street
Vallejo, CA 94590

Feingold Assn. of Visalia
3345 West Laurel Avenue
Visalia, CA 93277

COLORADO (Region 8)
Feingold Assn. of Colorado
7106 Maple Street
Longmont, CO 80501

CONNECTICUT (Region 1)
Connecticut Chapter of Feingold
   Assn. of the Merrimack Valley
4 Belinda Lane
Enfield, CT 06082

DELAWARE (Region 3)
Mid-Delaware Chapter of Feingold
   Assn. of Northern Delaware
Route 2, Box 486
Clayton, DE 19938

Feingold Assn. of Northern Delaware
2202 Lake Drive
Wilmington, DE 19808

**DISTRICT OF COLUMBIA
   (Region 3)**
Feingold Assn. of the Washington
   Area
P.O. Box 18116
Washington, D.C. 20021

FLORIDA (Region 4)
Feingold Assn. of Florida
P.O. Box 8460
Jacksonville, FL 32211

Orange Park Chapter of Feingold
   Assn. of Florida
2746 Holly Point R & W
Orange Park, FL 32073

GEORGIA (Region 4)
Feingold Assn. of Georgia
P.O. Box 28794
Atlanta, GA 30328

Chattahoochee Valley Feingold
   Assn.
Rt. 5, Box 536
Phenix City, AL 36867

GUAM (Region 9)
Regional Headquarters

HAWAII (Region 9)
Regional Headquarters

IDAHO (Region 10)
Area Representative of Feingold
   Assn. of the Northwest
P.O. Box 573
Osburn ID 83849

ILLINOIS (Region 5)
Feingold PATH of Illinois
5425 Maclaine Lane
Hanover Park, IL 60103

Southwestern Illinois Chapter of
   Feingold Assn. of Northern Illinois
319 E. Tanner
Waverly, IL 62692

Springfield Area Chapter of Fein-
   gold Assn. of Northern Illinois
P.O. Box 333
Williamsville, IL 62693

INDIANA (Region 5)

Bloomington Chapter of Feingold
Assn. of Indiana
2938 Ramble Road West
Bloomington, IN 47401

Northwest Indiana Chapter of
Feingold Assn. of Indiana
649 S. Main
Crown Point, IN 46307

Feingold Assn. of Indiana
8313 Scarsdale Court
Indianapolis, IN 46256

Muncie Chapter of Feingold Assn.
of America
Route 13, Box D-67
Muncie, IN 47302

Southwest Indiana Chapter of Feingold Assn. of Indiana
9977 Crestview Terrace
Newburgh, IN 47630

IOWA (Region 7)

Feingold Assn. of Iowa
P.O. Box 7112, Grand Avenue Sta-
tion
Des Moines, IA 50309

KANSAS (Region 7)

Feingold Assn. of Kansas
3200 S.E. Arbor Drive
Topeka, KS 66605

KENTUCKY (Region 4)

Feingold Assn. of Madisonville
Route 1
Manitou, KY 42436

LOUISIANA (Region 6)

Feingold Assn. of Louisiana
9272 Bermuda Avenue
Baton Rouge, LA 70810

Feingold Assn. of Baton Rouge
8945 Airline Highway
Baton Rouge, LA 70815

Feingold Assn. of Jennings Area
P.O. Box 1214
Jennings, LA 70546

Feingold Assn. of Metairie
1308 Colony Drive
Metairie, LA 70003

Feingold Assn. of Monroe Area
311 Paul Drive
West Monroe, LA 71291

MAINE (Region 1)

Portland Chapter of Feingold Assn.
of Merrimack Valley
29 Wolcott Street
Portland, ME 04102

MARYLAND (Region 3)

Southern Prince Georges County
Chapter of Feingold Assn. of the
Washington Area
6502 Acorn Court
Camp Springs, MD 20031

Calvert County Chapter of Fein-
gold Assn. of the Washington
Area
2616 Apple Way
R.R #1
Dunkirk, MD 20754

Harford County Chapter of Feingold Assn. of Northern Maryland
1818 Harewood Road
Edgewood, MD 21040

Montgomery County Chapter of
Feingold Assn. of the Washington Area
57 Midline Court
Gaithersburg, MD 20760

Northern Prince Georges County
Chapter of Feingold Assn. of the
Washington Area
4104 Beechwood Road
Hyattsville, MD 20782

St. Mary's/Charles County Chapter
of Feingold Assn. of the Washington Area
Rt. 2, Box 440
Mechanicsville, MD 20659

Feingold Assn. of Northern Maryland
2203 Springlake Drive
Timonium, MD 21093

MASSACHUSETTS (Region 1)
Plainville Chapter of Feingold
Assn. of Merrimack Valley
3 Birchwood Drive
Plainville, MA 02762

MICHIGAN (Region 5)
Alpena Chapter of Feingold Assn.
of Southeastern Michigan
525 Tawas
Alpena, MI 49707

Brighton Chapter of Feingold Assn.
of Southeastern Michigan
6530 Catalpa
Brighton, MI 48116

East Lansing/Okemus Chapter of
Feingold Assn. of Southeastern
Michigan
301 Highland
East Lansing, MI 48823

Fife Lake Chapter of Feingold
Assn. of Southeastern Michigan
Route 1 Box 166-D
Fife Lake, MI 49633

Frankenmuth Chapter of Feingold
Assn. of Southeastern Michigan
7136 S. Block Road
Frankenmuth, MI 48734

Lansing Area Chapter of Feingold
Assn. of Southeastern Michigan
9267 Looking Glassbrook Road
Grand Ledge, MI 48837

Grand Rapids Chapter of Feingold
Assn. of Southeastern Michigan
212 Saunders N.E.
Grand Rapids, MI 49505

Kalamazoo Chapter of Feingold
Assn. of Southeastern Michigan
1503 Academy
Kalamazoo, MI 49007

Lansing Chapter of Feingold Assn.
of Southeastern Michigan
224 Kenway
Lansing, MI 48917

Livonia Chapter of Feingold Assn.
of Southeastern Michigan
35220 W. Chicago
Livonia, MI 48150

Monroe Chapter of Feingold Assn.
of Southeastern Michigan
615 Parkwood Avenue
Monroe, MI 48161

Oak Park/Southfield/Birmingham
Chapter of Feingold Assn. of
Southeastern Michigan
15120 Oak Park Boulevard
Oak Park, MI 48237

Ortonville Chapter of Feingold
Assn. of Southeastern Michigan
5748 Honert
Ortonville, MI 48462

Saginaw Chapter of Feingold Assn.
of Southeastern Michigan
1706 Van Wagoner
Saginaw, MI 48603

Port Huron Chapter of Feingold
Assn. of Southeastern Michigan
516 N. 10th
St. Claire, MI 48079

Traverse City Chapter of Feingold
Assn. of Southeastern Michigan
742 High Lake Road
Traverse City, MI 49684

Feingold Assn. of Southeastern
Michigan
8691 Carriage Hill
Utica, MI 48087

MINNESOTA (Region 5)
Barnum Chapter of Feingold Assn.
of Minnesota
Route 2
Barnum, MN 55707

Feingold Assn. of Minnesota
6800 South Cedar Lake Road
Minneapolis, MN 55426

MISSISSIPPI (Region 4)
Regional Headquarters

MISSOURI (Region 7)
Feingold Assn. of Missouri
8007 E. 118th Street
Kansas City, MO 66605

MONTANA (Region 8)
Feingold Assn. of Montana
5925 Burnett Drive
Helena, MT 59601

Libby Chapter of Feingold Assn. of
Montana
Route 2, Box 846
Libby, MT 59923

NEBRASKA (Region 7)
Alliance Chapter of Feingold Assn.
of Omaha
916 W. 10th Street
Alliance, NB 69301

Feingold Assn. of Central Nebraska
105 W. Syria
Cairo, NB 68824

Lincoln Chapter of Feingold Assn.
of Omaha
6001 N. 14th Street
Lincoln, NB 68521

Feingold Assn. of Omaha
P.O. Box 37048
Omaha, NB 68137

NEVADA (Region 9)
Regional Headquarters

NEW HAMPSHIRE (Region 1)
Regional Headquarters

NEW JERSEY (Region 2)
Feingold Assn. of Central New Jersey
60-A Warren Drive
Edison, NJ 08817

Feingold Assn. of Gloucester
112 Villanova Road
Glassboro, NJ 08028

Feingold Assn. of Burlington
County
P.O. Box 528
Marlton, NJ 08053

NEW MEXICO (Region 6)
Regional Headquarters

NEW YORK (Region 2)
Feingold Assn. of Buffalo & Erie
County
P.O. Box 32
Amherst, NY 14226

Baldwinsville Chapter of Feingold
Assn. of Central New York
2268 Connell Terrace
Baldwinsville, NY 13027

Liverpool Chapter of Feingold
Assn. of Central New York
105 Beechwood Avenue
Liverpool, NY 13088

Feingold Assn. of Capital District
P.O. Box 11670
Loudonville, NY 12211

Feingold Assn. of New York
1652 Baker Avenue
Merrick, NY 11566

Feingold Assn. of Mid-Hudson
Valley
35 South Gate Drive
Poughkeepsie, NY 12601

Feingold Assn. of Monroe County
P.O. Box 4716
Rochester, NY 14612

Feingold Assn. of New York
1034 Jericho Turnpike
Smithtown, NY 11787

NORTH CAROLINA (Region 4)
Feingold Assn. of Charlotte
3224 Lazy Branch Road
Matthews, NC 28105

NORTH DAKOTA (Region 8)
Regional Headquarters

OHIO (Region 5)
Feingold Assn. of North Central
Ohio
1058 Columbus Circle S.
Ashland, OH 44805

Feingold Assn. of Southern Ohio
15455 Winchester Road
Ashville, OH 43103

OKLAHOMA (Region 6)
Feingold Assn. of Tulsa
P.O. Box 3493
Tulsa, OK 74101

OREGON (Region 10)
Area Representative of Feingold
Assn of the Northwest
8845 S.W. Rebecca Lane
Beaverton, OR 97005

Area Representative of Feingold
Assn. of the Northwest
60239 Tall Pine Avenue
Bend, OR 97701

Area Representative of Feingold
Assn. of the Northwest
1100 N.E. 13th Circle
Canby, OR 97013

Area Representative of Feingold
Assn. of the Northwest
37100 Resort Drive
Cloverdale, OR 97112

Eugene Representative of Feingold
Assn. of the Northwest
333 Van Avenue
Eugene, OR 97401

Springfield Representative of Feingold Assn. of the Northwest
1205 Lake Drive
Eugene, OR 97404

Area Representative of Feingold
Assn. of the Northwest
Route 3, Box 26
McMinnville, OR 97128

Area Representative of Feingold
Assn. of the Northwest
3516 N.E. Riverside
Pendleton, OR 97801

Area Representative of Feingold
Assn. of the Northwest
Route 1, Box 690
Rainier, OR 97048

Salem Representative of Feingold
Assn. of the Northwest
8106 Sunnyside Road S.E.
Salem, OR 97302

Area Representative of Feingold
Assn. of the Northwest
303 S.W. 4th
Scappoose, OR 97056

Medford Representative of Feingold
Assn. of the Northwest
1045 Beeson Lane
Talent, OR 97540

Area Representative of Feingold
Assn. of the Northwest
14885 S.W. Sunrise Lane
Tigard, OR 97223

PENNSYLVANIA (Region 3)
Lackawana County Affiliate of
Feingold Assn. of Philadelphia
and Surrounding Counties
537 Gladiola Drive
Clarks Summit, PA 18411

Dingmans Ferry Chapter of Fein-
gold Assn. of Pike County
Blue Heron Lake
Dingmans Ferry, PA 18328

Feingold Assn. of Greensburg
117 Sherwood Drive
Greensburg, PA 15601

Feingold Assn. of Lehigh Valley
P.O. Box 175
Hellertown, PA 18055

Berks County Chapter of Feingold
Assn. of Lehigh Valley
707 E. Walnut Street
Kutztown, PA 19530

Feingold Assn. of Lancaster
County
P.O. Box 44
Landisville, PA 17538

Feingold Assn. of Pike County
606 W. Harford Street
Milford, PA 18337

Feingold Assn. of Philadelphia &
Surrounding Counties
3439 Chalfont Drive
Philadelphia, PA 19154

Feingold Assn. of Western Pennsylvania
133 Painter Street
Trafford, PA 15085

Feingold Assn. of West Chester
1156 Kingsway Road, #6
West Chester, PA 19380

PUERTO RICO (Region 2)
Regional Headquarters

RHODE ISLAND (Region 1)
Cumberland Chapter of Feingold
  Assn. of the Merrimack Valley
29 Nicholas Drive
Cumberland, RI 02864

Tiverton Chapter of Feingold Assn.
  of the Merrimack Valley
100 Peaceful Way
Tiverton, RI 02878

SOUTH CAROLINA (Region 4)
Feingold Assn. of South Carolina
330 Hillsborough Drive
Greenville, SC 29615

SOUTH DAKOTA (Region 8)
Feingold Assn. of South Dakota
Route #1
Agar, SD 57520

TENNESSEE (Region 4)
Feingold Assn. of Memphis
110 South Front Street
Memphis, TN 38103

TEXAS (Region 6)
Feingold Assn. of Dallas-Ft. Worth
  Metroplex
P.O. Box 13007
Arlington, TX 76013

Feingold Assn. of Austin
1400 The High Road
Austin, TX 78746

Feingold Assn. of Baytown
P.O. Box 7047
Baytown, TX 77520

Feingold Assn. of Brownsville
925 Los Ebanos
Brownsville, TX 78520

Feingold Assn. of El Paso
5549 Sarah Anne
El Paso, TX 79924

Feingold Assn. of Houston
3219 Fondren
Houston, TX 77063

Feingold Assn. of Central Texas
1503 Mockingbird Lane
Kileen, TX 76541

UTAH (Region 8)
American Fork Chapter of Feingold
  Assn. of Utah
195 West 700 North
American Fork, UT 84003

Bountiful Chapter of Feingold
  Assn. of Utah
935 North 325 West
Bountiful, UT 84010

Clearfield Chapter of Feingold
  Assn. of Utah
893 Birch
Clearfield, UT 84015

Feingold Assn. of Utah
P.O. Box 25726
Salt Lake City, UT 84125

Salt Lake City Chapter of Feingold
  Assn. of Utah
1428 Lombardy Circle
Salt Lake City, UT 84121

VERMONT (Region 1)
Regional Headquarters

VIRGIN ISLANDS (Region 2)
Regional Headquarters

VIRGINIA (Region 3)
Fairfax County Chapter of Feingold Assn. of the Washington Area
2502 Davis Avenue
Alexandria, VA 22302

Washington, D.C. Chapter of Feingold Assn. of the Washington Area
1925 Stonebridge Road
Alexandria, VA 22304

Charlottesville Chapter of Feingold Assn. of the Washington Area
P.O. Box 90
Batesville, VA 22924

Norfolk Chapter of Feingold Assn. of the Washington Area
1200 Meredith Place
Norfolk, VA 23505

Peninsula Chapter of Feingold Assn. of the Washington Area
248 Cedar Road
Poquoson, VA 23662

Richmond Area Feingold Assn.
1009 Elaine Avenue
Richmond, VA 23235

Feingold Assn. of Roanoke Valley
P.O. Box 3044
Roanoke, VA 24015

WASHINGTON (Region 10)
Area Representative of Feingold Assn. of the Northwest
12014 N.E. 65th
Kirkland, WA 98033

Area Representative of Feingold Assn. of the Northwest
3035 S Genesee Street
Seattle, WA 98108

Area Representative of Feingold Assn. of the Northwest
W. 1121—6th Avenue
Spokane, WA 99204

Area Representative of Feingold Assn. of the Northwest
623 North "C" Street
Tacoma, WA 98403

WASHINGTON D.C. (REGION 3)
(See *District of Columbia*)

WEST VIRGINIA (Region 3)
Charleston Chapter of Feingold Assn. of the Washington Area
1568 Smith Road
Charleston, WV 25314

Clarksburg Chapter of Feingold Assn. of the Washington Area
General Delivery
West Milford, WV 26451

WISCONSIN (Region 5)
Hudson Chapter of Feingold Assn. of Minnesota
405 Locust Street
Hudson, WI 54016

WYOMING (Region 8)
Regional Headquarters

Appendix VI

Associations for Children with Learning Disabilities (ACLD)

(State affiliates as of March, 1980)

NATIONAL HEADQUARTERS
ACLD, 4156 Library Road
Pittsburgh, PA 15234

OUTSIDE UNITED STATES:
Canada: Canadian ACLD
Kildare House, 323 Chapel Street
Ottawa, Ontario K1N 7Z2

Quebec ACLD
4820 Van Horne Avenue, Suite 8
Montreal, Quebec H3W 1J3

ALABAMA
P.O. Box 11588
Montgomery AL 36111

ALASKA
7420 Old Harbor Avenue
Anchorage, Ak 99504

ARIZONA
P.O. Box 15525
Phoenix, AZ 85060

ARKANSAS
2500 N. Tyler
P.O. Box 7316
Little Rock, AR 72217

CALIFORNIA
(California Assn. for Neurologically Handicapped Children)
P.O. Box 61067
Sacramento, CA 95860

COLORADO
P.O. Box 10535
University Park Station
Denver, CO 80210

CONNECTICUT
Connecticut Assn. for Children with Perceptual Learning Disabilities
20 Raymond Road
West Hartford, CT 06107

DELAWARE
(Diamond State ACLD)
15 Barnard Street
Newark, DE 19711

DISTRICT OF COLUMBIA
2899 Audubon Terrace N.W.
Washington, D.C. 20008

FLORIDA
2766 Banchory Road
Winter Park, FL 32792

GEORGIA
P.O. Box 29492
Atlanta, GA 30329

HAWAII
200 N. Vineyard Boulevard, #402
Honolulu, HI 96817

242

IDAHO
5217 Wylie Lane
Boise, ID 83703 ᵢ

ILLINOIS
P.O. Box A-3239
Chicago, IL 60690

INDIANA
51416 Orange Road
South Bend, IN 46628

IOWA
2819 48th Street
Des Moines, IA 50310

KANSAS
114 West 8th Street, Suite #4
Topeka, KS 66601

KENTUCKY
1323 South 3rd Street
Louisville, KY 40208

LOUISIANA
P.O. Box 205
Tioga, LA 71477

MAINE
P.O.Box 93
West Southport, ME 04576

MARYLAND
Route 2, Box 2362-B
La Plata, MD 20646

MASSACHUSETTS
(Massachusetts CHILD)
P.O. Box 261
Chestnut Hill, MA 02167

(Blue Hills ACLD)
154 West Street
Randolph, MA 02368

MICHIGAN
20777 Randall
Farmington Hills, MI 48024

MINNESOTA
1821 University Avenue
Rm 494-N
St. Paul, Minnesota 55104

MISSISSIPPI
P.O. Box 12083
Jackson, MS 39211

MISSOURI
P.O. Box 3303
Glenstone Station
Springfield, MO 65804

MONTANA
511 Burlington
Billings, MT 59101

NEBRASKA
P.O. Box 6464
Omaha, NE 68106

NEW HAMPSHIRE
815 Elm Street
Manchester, N.H. 03101

NEW JERSEY
P.O. Box 249
Convent Station, NJ 07961

NEW MEXICO
7021 Prospect Place N.E.
Albuquerque, NM 87110

NEW YORK
(New York Association for the
  Learning Disabled)
217 Lark Street
Albany, NY 12210

NEVADA
6208 South El Camino Road
Las Vegas, NV 89121

NORTH CAROLINA
2204 Market Street
Wilmington, NC 28403

NORTH DAKOTA
1866 South Grandview Lane
Bismark, ND 58501

OHIO
4601 North High Street
Columbus, OH 43214

OKLAHOMA
3701 N.W. 62nd Street
Oklahoma City, OK 73112

OREGON
1133 S.W. Market Street, Rm. 202
Portland, OR 97201

PENNSYLVANIA
1383 Arcadia Road
Lancaster, PA 17601

PUERTO RICO
11-19 Salamanca
Torrimar Guaynabo, PR 00657

RHODE ISLAND
P.O. Box 6685
Providence, RI 02904

SOUTH CAROLINA
608 Hatrick Road
Columbia, SC 29209

SOUTH DAKOTA
1605 South Tenth Avenue
Sioux Falls, SD 57105

TENNESSEE
101 Stanton Lane
Oak Ridge, TN 37830

TEXAS
1011 West 31st Street
Austin, TX 78705

UTAH
4180 Mackay
Taylorsville, UT 05602

VERMONT
9 Heaton Street
Montpelier, VT 05602

VIRGINIA
3851 North Upland Street
Arlington, VA 22207

WASHINGTON
444 N.E. Ravenna Boulevard, Rm.
  206
Seattle, WA 98115

WASHINGTON D.C.
(see *District of Columbia*)

WEST VIRGINIA
1931 Seventh Avenue
St. Albans, WV 25177

WISCONSIN
922 E. Fillmore
Eau Claire, WI 54701

WYOMING
710 Gerald Place
Laramie, WY 82070

INDEX

8